T0130515

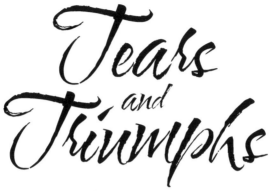

Tears and Triumphs

A Memoir of a Breast Cancer Journey
with Two Perspectives

Caroline Logan
with
Martin Logan

BALBOA.
PRESS
A DIVISION OF HAY HOUSE

Balboa Press books may be ordered through booksellers or by contacting:

Balboa Press
A Division of Hay House
1663 Liberty Drive
Bloomington, IN 47403
www.balboapress.com.au
1 (877) 407-4847

Print information available on the last page.

ISBN: 978-1-5043-1649-1 (sc)
ISBN: 978-1-5043-1650-7 (e)

Balboa Press rev. date: 01/16/2019

Contents

Dedication

For Martin, for your constant and unwavering love, support, humour and strength. I love you.

For Jade and Tyson, for always sticking together when times are tough-love you guys.

For my Mum, love you mummy-bear.

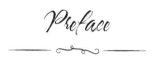

Preface

Finally, after 3 years, I have put fingers to keyboard and written this memoir! I now see the delay in writing was really the impact this disease had on me and my inability until now, to actually relive the experience.

This book was written to tell my story and that of my family and how the experience of a Breast Cancer diagnosis affected our lives.

It is a deeply personal and at times very open account of the choices we made, the result of those choices and how they impacted and still continue to impact our lives.

For those on the outer, the journey may sometimes seem significantly shorter. Diagnosis, treatment, finished. For those traversing the course on a daily basis, living with the uncertainty, fear, pain, tears, and choices - the road is so much longer.

I want this book to be passed around, given to a family member, offered to a friend or bought for a colleague, so that our experience can inspire, support, educate or enlighten someone who has had a diagnosis.

Dear reader, help is out there, sometimes you will find it in the most amazing places and from those you didn't even know existed!

Acknowledgements

Firstly, thank you to the team at Balboa Press for their constant and timely support, without which this memoir would not have been published. The time was finally right Al!

A huge round of applause and sincere gratitude to my amazing proof reader Gillean Logan, whose support and words of encouragement have meant more to me than she will ever know.

A big heartfelt thank you to the following people and organisations, on behalf of myself and my family; The staff and volunteers at Sir Charles Gairdner Hospital, Subiaco – especially Dr. Kallyani Ponniah and Dr. Roshi Kamyab - who helped make the journey a whole lot easier with their care, empathy and professionalism and all the staff who work at the Breast Centre for their constant attention and unceasing guidance - also, the volunteer ladies who offer a nice hot cuppa when you need it the most.

Also, Breast Cancer Care W.A. for providing W.A. women ourselves included - free of charge, the resources that are needed at such a hard time – a special mention to Moira Waters, without who my initial confusion and shock at the diagnosis and treatment regime would have been so much harder to process and accept.

Thanks to the Zonta International Volunteers - for the amazing breast cushions.

And definitely not forgetting Berlei – for supplying free of charge the My Care Kit, which contains the post-surgery bra and padded foam form, which start to make you feel whole again.

Chapter 1

Diagnosis

If my story has to have a starting place, where it all began, then it really began back in 2004, after having my regular Pap smear and health check. The results showed cellular changes. After having treatment (a cone biopsy which involved having the inside of my cervix cauterised) for these changes known as CIN 1, I decided that from now on, I would have a yearly pap smear. The doctor who I had been seeing for many years, had always included a breast examination during my annual visit.

On May 6th, 2013, I had my annual health check appointment. After the doctor checked my moles, she asked me to lay on the exam table and lift my arms behind my head. She then proceeded to perform a breast examination, making small circular movements around the right breast (as we're told and shown on all the brochures) and as she came to the base of my breast, she stopped and made a comment that she thought she could feel a small lump. I was asked to stand up and she again felt the breast and asked me to do the same and sure enough, I could feel a lump, shaped like a ladyfinger grape, so clearly.

How could I have missed this?!

My doctor announced that she would refer me for a mammogram, an ultrasound and possibly a fine needle aspiration (FNA). She advised me to make the booking as soon as possible. I also had to have a mole removed, as the doctor didn't like the look of it. I remember leaving the surgery and standing on the grass outside the building.

"Well, that wasn't a very nice time that's for sure. I had a pap smear, have to have a mole cut off AND I have a grape-sized lump in my breast," I said to myself.

I made an appointment for the mammogram etc. the following day, and had to wait a week! Well, that week seemed more like a month. If you've ever had to wait for important news, then you'll know exactly how I felt.

When the day finally arrived for my

mammogram appointment, it happened to coincide with my doctor's visit for the removal of the mole, later in the afternoon.

In the morning, I attended the radiography clinic and was asked to go to a cubicle and undress and put on the lovely blue robe that they have for you. After a five minute wait, I was guided into the room where the mammography machine was. The female technician was really nice and friendly and tried to put me at ease, which is quite a job when your breast is being squished in between two metal plates! It didn't hurt though, more uncomfortable than anything, like having to cuddle a big metal machine while it does things to your breasts. The mammogram probably took about thirty minutes and then I was asked to wait for about ten minutes while the technician checked the pictures. She returned and took me back to the cubicle and asked me to wait.

The next technician took me to another room and asked me to lie on the table. She was going to perform the ultrasound examination. It's quite a strange environment, as it's really quiet in the room, except for the blips that the machine makes when the technician takes a picture, and no-one is saying anything to you, so you don't have any idea of what they're seeing, and basically you're trying not to freak out.

The technician seemed to be going over the same spots on my breast quite a few times and she finally told me that she would have to perform an Ultrasound-guided Fine Needle Aspiration (FNA). This is where a fine needle is inserted into the lump/s and a small piece of tissue is extracted for biopsy. I had three places in my right breast at ten o'clock, two o'clock and six o'clock where tissue was taken. The procedure was not the most comfortable I must say, but obviously necessary, so I was trying not to be a baby. I did come out with a few bruises a day later though. Little did I know, they would be my first battle scars.

An FNA is a procedure where a fine needle is inserted into the lump/s and a small piece of tissue is extracted for biopsy. To start an FNA examination, the skin of your breast is washed with antiseptic. A thin needle (similar to a needle used for taking a blood sample), is placed through the skin into the breast, to sample the area of interest under the guidance of an ultrasound. The needle stays in the breast for a short time, while it is gently moved back and forth to enable cells to be collected.

Later that afternoon I headed to my doctor's appointment to have the mole removed. As my doctor was readying me for the procedure, she asked how the tests that day had gone. I told her they were fine, a little painful but ok. She then floored me by telling me some news.

"They're worried."

"Sorry?" I asked.

My doctor then told me that the radiology clinic had already contacted her and said they were worried about the images they had seen on the mammogram and ultrasound and as soon as they had the test results back they would call her. I was told the results should be in by Friday morning, three days from now. What a wait!

After I left the surgery that afternoon, I decided then and there, that I wanted to be calm. I have heard other people say that they're going to "fight cancer", and people often say that a person put up a good fight. I felt quite the opposite. I didn't want to 'fight'. I wanted to stay calm and peaceful and just move through the experience in a balanced way if that was a possibility. I asked God to help me through whatever was going to come and to please put those in my path that could help me. I could only do it with his help.

I told my husband Martin what I had decided and he agreed with me. We would go through whatever was going to come in as peaceful a way as possible.

The morning finally came to visit my doctor to get the results. I arrived early to the surgery and was sitting outside in the carpark in my car when my mobile phone rang. It was my mum. She asked where I was and I told her. I asked her where she was and she said she was also in the carpark! I felt a bit niggled as I had just wanted to be peaceful and calm and truthfully to be on my own, but I know my ma! I asked her if she wanted to come into the surgery with me.

"Yes!" was her grateful reply.

We were called into the doctor's office and she told us that she hadn't received the results yet. She made a phone call and was told the pathology lab was extremely busy and they would try to get the results as soon as possible. It was very frustrating having to wait all weekend not knowing anything.

To make matters worse, we were tiptoeing around the house with our possible news. My daughter Jade was doing her Year twelve TEE exams and we didn't want to distract her unnecessarily, so Martin and I used to talk in the bathroom, and when I spoke to my mum on the phone, we shut the bedroom door and talked in code, it was just like when the kids were little and had learnt to spell!

To support myself during the wait, I used my Pomanders. In 2000, I had studied the Aura-Soma© colour system and still had a set. The Pomanders are used through the aura and contain herbs and essences to provide protection and support. They are my "go to" whenever I feel extra support is needed on any level.

On Monday 20th May 2013, I was standing in my bedroom getting ready for work when my mobile phone rang. I answered it and heard my doctors' voice. She said she had the results back from the biopsy. My heart stopped, as she told me without a doubt, I had malignant breast cancer in the right breast.

I couldn't think and I think I stopped breathing as well. All of the things I wanted to see and do in my life came into my mind all at once. I wanted to see my kids grow up and get married and have babies. I wanted to grow old and wrinkly with my hubby. I certainly didn't want to leave all that behind, until I was a ripe old age. I think I went into shock and tried to get my head around the news as the doctor continued speaking. She told me she would pass on all my results and personal details to the Breast Clinic at Sir Charles Gairdner Hospital (SCGH) in Nedlands, W.A. and that I would hear from them as soon as possible.

I received a letter from the hospital letting me know my first appointment was booked for 5th June 2013.

The first person I called after hearing the devastating news was my husband Martin. He then proceeded to go into denial and stayed there for about a month! I had to let his side of the family know our news, as he just couldn't face it, let alone voice it. Later in this chapter, Martin will tell you how he felt about the diagnosis.

I then called my mum Marie, brother John and sister Julia and they all took the news as well as can be expected. There were a lot of "Oh's," and "What can we do's?" John talked a bit about an alternative treatment that a friend of his was trying for cancer, but I just explained that as this was my life we were dealing with, I was going to do exactly as the doctors suggested. I believe in and have personally used some alternative treatments, but this was not going to be one of those times.

My next phone call was to my manager. I was working part-time as a foreign exchange teller and had only been in the role since January. He couldn't have been more supportive and caring. The next day he came to see me at the store and gave me a big hug and let me know that he had talked to the owners of the company. They had decided whatever I needed to do for myself in regard to treatment etc, they were right behind me and would support me one hundred per cent. This was great news as we didn't know how much this experience would cost us at that time. I was honest and said that I didn't know what treatment would be involved, but I would keep them updated every step of the way. I wanted to continue working as long as possible.

Telling my good friend Rachelle, was something I should have done a different way, now that I think about it. We used to meet about once a month to catch up on family gossip and just natter and laugh for the entire time at Dome, usually around three hours. On this particular visit I had some news for her which I had decided to tell her after our visit, but before my daughter, Jade arrived from work. As we hadn't told the children yet, I wanted to tell Rachelle without Jade being there.

So we were enjoying our visit as always and towards the end Jade sent me a message that she had finished work and was heading across the road to Dome, to come home with me. So, I quickly told Rachelle I had some news. She actually looked a bit excited. Poor thing.

"I've got breast cancer," I said.

She looked at me for a minute. I think she was trying to see if I was telling her some sick joke. I then had to quickly explain the situation so far, not giving the poor girl any time to digest the news. We had known each other for about ten years at that stage. I should have put myself in her shoes and thought better about how to tell her. I could see Jade coming closer to the building so I had to talk fast. I said everything I wanted her to know, and when Jade walked in I was all smiles again. We said our goodbyes with lots of hugs and kisses, and then I left my poor friend to mull over the news I had just blurted to her. Sorry, Rachelle, I apologise for the way I told you.

In W.A. the Cancer Council of W.A. have some excellent resources available free of charge to help you when breaking the news of a diagnosis.

They also have resources for family and friends to learn helpful ways to offer assistance. So when telling your loved ones or even work colleagues, please be mindful of your timing and the circumstances and environment you tell them in. It just may help them in the long run. I found during this experience that help sometimes came from a direction I didn't expect. As we all handle a crisis in different ways, those you expect much from, may not be able to give, and those you don't expect anything from, pop up out of the blue to offer assistance.

Martin and I made a conscious decision to delay telling my children Jade, then seventeen and Tyson fifteen, until we had had the appointment for the Breast Centre. By this time Jade had finished her first round of exams. For me, this was the hardest thing I had to do. I felt it should be a family affair, so I asked my mum to come over and Martin and I were present as well.

I asked Tyson to come into the lounge room, as Jade was about to finish studying in another room. As she walked by the lounge room I asked her if she would come into the room. She was about to bolt, so I moved in front of her to stop her. When Jade was six, her father and I divorced,

Martin is their stepfather. Jade told me later, this was why she was trying to run, she thought that something similar was happening again. We explained to her that it was nothing like that, we just had some news to tell.

So with the children seated and their nanna and Martin there for support, I began to tell my beautiful children that I had recently had a doctors check-up and that the doctor had found a lump in my breast.

Jade asked, "Is it cancer?"

I looked at them both and replied "Yes."

My children's faces crumbled a bit, as did my heart and they looked towards Martin and their nanna for their reactions. To ease their shock and bring about some positivity into the situation, I let them know straight away that the doctor has said she believed it was caught early, so it was called Early Stage breast cancer. These words were my Hope, I was pinning my life on them. I wanted the children to have that hope as well.

I sat on the lounge and my seventeen-year-old baby girl came and cuddled me. Jade was looking up into my eyes with her beautiful blue eyes, as she had so many times in her life.

"Are you going to die?" she asked me.

The tears are streaming down my face as I write these words now, as I can still see the pain in her eyes, as she wondered if her mum was going to live or not.

My words to her were "I really don't know, but from what the doctor says, it was caught early which gives me a good chance and that's what we have to hold on to baby." Jade knew my regular doctor and that fact seemed to help her and enabled her to trust the doctor's words that her mum would be alright. I think my doctor is Jade's hero!

My son Tyson, being the thinker, had had a few moments to think about things and had been having a quiet word to nanna. He then asked what the doctors were going to do, and I let him know what a great question that was to ask. I said that they would possibly have to remove the breast with cancer in it. He pondered that for a moment before asking what would happen then.

I looked at Martin and then said: "Mum gets new boobs, yay!"

Well, that got us all laughing. I really believe the children coped as well as they did because they could see us supporting each other. We let them know if they had any questions about anything they could ask. Considering the news they had just been given, Jade and Tyson took it all in their stride and coped really well. They had always been the best kids and hadn't given me any grief. During the whole experience, they just continued on with their lives and got on with things. I'm very proud of them both for their courage and tenacity during this very difficult period. My kids were tougher than I knew.

I made sure I informed the kids' school so they would have support while they were there, and it was an amazing time, with prayers being said for me and words of encouragement for our family in the school newsletter. I also let the kids know they could tell their friends if they wanted to, it was totally up to them. Jade told most of her friends and teachers and they all gave her wonderful support and a shoulder to cry on if she needed it. Tyson also told a couple of friends and his teachers were also very supportive and accommodating. By the way, Jade passed all of her exams!

I had two uncles living in Melbourne at the time and breaking the news to them and their families was a bit hard. My father Bill had passed away from cancer in 2011, so it was still a bit raw for all of us. They were extremely supportive and sent well wishes and asked me to keep them informed along the way. Sadly, both of those lovely uncles have also passed now, Uncle Ray after heart complications following surgery for a recurrence of mouth cancer and Uncle Brian from lung cancer.

During the weeks we had to wait for the appointment to the Breast Clinic at S.C.G.H, I tried to educate myself as much as I could, and I believe that's how I came to grips with the diagnosis. I felt that if I knew what was going to happen I could make informed decisions about treatments etc. I had learnt from my time at uni, not to trust any old website, so I went straight on to the BCNA (Breast Cancer Network Australia) website and started looking around. I didn't know at this time, what stage of breast cancer I had.

These stages are 0-4 and are determined by the size of the breast cancer present and where the cancer is found in the body. Treatment options can be discussed relating to the stage of breast cancer found.

While I was looking around the BCNA website, I noticed a small link that reads "My

Journey Kit." I clicked on the link and was taken to a page that talked about this amazing resource and how it could be ordered. It was free of charge and was sent to me within a couple of days.

This resource is invaluable! If you or someone you know has breast cancer please, please order this kit.

When I received the kit I opened it right away. It contained an Information Guide booklet which was divided up into sections relating to things such as diagnosis, choosing treatment options, living with breast cancer and life after treatment. There was a CD called "When the woman you love has early breast cancer." My kit also contained a Guide for Women with Early breast cancer booklet which also had invaluable information. Every night I would sit in bed and read. These resources helped me to choose what treatment and reconstruction options I had. And truthfully, the knowledge the books gave me, took away some of the fear of the unknown. I felt better arming myself with knowledge. I started to understand what might come down the road, and maybe how to handle it.

Martin and I started talking about the

possibility that I may need a mastectomy. I'm not sure why, but for some reason, we both just felt that would be the outcome. I would tell him about topics that were written in the booklets and we would talk about them. He couldn't really bring himself to read them himself but that was okay with me.

My gorgeous husband used to say "As long as I have you, I don't mind what they do."

I remember one night I was reading through the booklets in bed, while Martin read his own book beside me. I was reading about Nipple reconstruction and read that you can buy stick-on nipples. Well, to say we laughed was an understatement! Then came all the naughty jokes about getting them stuck in your mouth etc. you know what I mean I'm sure. It felt so good to be able to laugh together about what was to come. We were seeing that we could still laugh and be happy, even though we had some rough times ahead.

Inside the Information guide booklet, some women briefly share their own experiences, but often I found that I couldn't read them. It upset me too much. I just read factual information and found that was the easiest way for me to cope.

The last but definitely not least booklet I received in the Kit was a My Journey 'Personal Record' booklet. I cannot express how much this booklet helped me throughout my breast cancer experience and still continues to help me as I write this memoir.

My Personal Record booklet was divided up into seven sections: Personal, Appointments, Treatment, Personal reflections / Journal, Professional support / Contacts, Calendar / Medical & Treatment Expenses. I was able to fill these pages, and boy I did, with lots of useful information about myself. I probably used the personal, calendar and journal pages more than any others.

The pages allowed me to write down any questions I had, my appointment times and dates, which was especially good for surgery times and post-op appointments. There was also room for writing how I felt after my treatments and information that was discussed with my doctors during visits.

At times, there is a lot to take in and to be able to jot down important information and have it all in one place later, when you are more able to take it in, was an absolute godsend.

From time to time within the following chapters, I will add excerpts from my journal. They are deeply personal and I'm happy to be sharing them with you, to offer you an insight into what went on 'behind the scenes'.

The My Journey Kit is available to order from the BCNA website and is available as I received it in 2013 and now also in a downloadable format. Take note though, I have recently been told by staff (April 2018) at BCNA that the 'Personal Record' booklet is not available with the downloaded version of the kit.

During the time I was waiting for my appointment to SCGH breast clinic, my mind kept thinking about a lady called Sue who is a friend of a friend of mine, who I had met and known about twenty years ago. Sue was the only person I had known that had been diagnosed with breast cancer. Her treatment involved a mastectomy. As I mentioned earlier, I had asked God to put people in my path that would help me. All I wanted to do was to talk to Sue, as I felt she would give me much needed support and information. About a week later my wish came true.

One morning, as I was working with my

colleague Peng at the foreign exchange shop, who should walk in the door but Sue! I was gobsmacked, to say the least. I went out the office door and gave her a big hug.

"I don't believe you're here, I've wanted to talk to you so badly and now here you are," I said excitedly.

I quickly explained my diagnosis and we had a quick chat. Sue seemed to be in a hurry as she was meeting someone for coffee. I asked her if I could catch up with her later in the week.

"I'm sorry," she said, "We're going home tomorrow, so I can't meet with you."

I didn't realise what she was saying as I thought she lived in Perth.

"What do you mean, where do you live?" I asked her.

Now, please believe me when you read the next lines, as I am NOT telling fibs as God is my witness.

Sue replied to me "We live in Inner Mongolia." What!!!! Sue's husband had been working there for a few years.

Peng and I looked at each other and laughed. I told Sue how I had been thinking so much about her and wanting to somehow get in touch and then here she was, standing in front of me, and had come all the way from Inner Mongolia.

I really wanted to continue our conversation, so I asked Sue if I could have her email address, and we swapped them then and there. Sue said I could email her anytime and ask anything I liked, which gave me great feelings of support. Sue hurried away leaving Peng and me with the feeling that there were definitely greater powers at work here than we would ever know.

About three hours later, who should walk into the shop again but Sue. She walked up to my window and handed me a business card.

"This is my friend who I met when I was diagnosed with breast cancer and she helped me a lot. She can put you in touch with many people who can help you and she's waiting for your call this afternoon."

I couldn't believe it. My heart swelled with joy. I was hoping that God wasn't playing with me. I rushed out and gave Sue a big hug and thanked her and told her I would definitely contact her friend. Her friend's name is Ros Worthington and she is the founder of Breast Cancer Care WA.

Breast Cancer Care WA is a WA charity that provides personalised emotional, practical and financial support and care to people affected by breast cancer. This wonderful W.A. charity receives no government funding and is solely supported financially by the public of W.A.

I called Ros later in the day and she told me that her organisation could help me and that they would be there every step of the way. Whether getting to an appointment, someone to talk to, helping with shopping, cooking, cleaning or paying a bill, help was available.

To say this organisation helped us, is really to minimise what they did for us. It went way beyond helping. I will tell you more about how this unbelievable organisation and its wonderful people helped us throughout the coming chapters.

When the appointment day finally came (written in my Personal Record Calendar) to attend the breast clinic at SCGH, Martin and I went along not knowing what to expect. We had been trying not to freak out over the past few weeks but the wait was finally over. Martin's boss had been very understanding in giving him the day off to attend the appointment. Please take someone with you when you go to your first appointment, as there is a lot of talking done and you may have questions that you want to ask.

Martin and I arrived at the Breast Clinic reception and I had to tell the lady my name and she ticked me off her list. She then wrote my details on a coloured card and asked me to go around the corner into the waiting room and put my card into the corresponding coloured plastic holder. As time goes on you get different coloured cards, depending on which stage of the journey you are at. We did as she asked and took a seat.

As we all hear, Australian statistics now show that one in eight women will develop breast cancer by the age of eighty-five. The outcome of these statistics can be seen in the waiting room at the Breast Clinic. If I can impart any words of wisdom regarding the Breast Centre and its appointments, it is to do the following things:

- Take a book
- Take a snack
- Stay calm
- Take a friend
- Stay calm
- Take a pen and paper or ask your friend to, to write down anything that you think of.
- Have your questions ready to ask the doctor. They're very busy and it's good to

23

keep the flow of patients going. You don't want to be the last one of the day!
- Take change for the carpark.

These things will help you during these clinic visits. Remember just because you have a time specified on the appointment letter, doesn't mean this is the time you will see the doctor. Sometimes things happen unexpectedly and through no one's fault. We often had delays in appointment times, but after a couple of visits, we began to be at ease with the wait.

My name was finally called so Martin and I followed the doctor into the clinic room. The doctor's name was Dr Roshi Kamyab. We were also joined in the room by a McGrath Breast care nurse.

I sat at the table next to the doctor and Martin sat across from me on another chair. Dr Kamyab introduced herself and the breast care nurse. We discussed the findings of the FNA and the Mammogram which I had earlier in May. She told me that it was very clear that I had a malignant invasive tumour Stage two, approx. 20mm in the right breast. This means that the cancer cells were not contained and had spread to the surrounding breast tissue. I also had what is termed as Ductal Carcinoma In Situ (DCIS).

DCIS is referred to as non-invasive cancer. This meant that there were cancer cells present, however, they were contained within the milk ducts of my right breast.

After the initial diagnosis was given, Dr Kamyab said she needed me to have a couple more tests done. The right breast results were quite clear but there were still areas that needed further investigation. The left breast mammogram and FNA showed inconclusive results. I would need to have further Core Biopsies taken from the left and right breasts. Dr Kamyab said that at this stage, her recommendation would be the removal of the lump and probably radiation treatment. We would have a clearer picture once the test results came back.

A Core needle biopsy is a procedure to remove a small amount of suspicious tissue from the breast with a larger core or hollow needle. The procedure is usually performed under local anaesthetic to the area involved.

Dr Kamyab made me an appointment to return to the Breast Clinic on Friday 7th June 2013 to have the further tests done. We would then return to discuss treatment options. Martin and I thanked her and left the Breast Clinic. We still didn't have a precise treatment plan but at least we were on our way. We were trying to think as positively as we could. I told Martin that as the tests may take a while, I would be quite happy to go to the appointment on my own.

I made my way to the Breast Clinic on the appointed Friday. I was a little bit nervous, but I was really just glad that something was being done. I checked in with the ladies at reception and took my coloured card around to the waiting area.

My name was finally called and I was taken through to another area where mammograms and other tests are done. I was asked to undress and put a robe on in the change room. I was then taken into a clinic room for the ultrasound-guided Core Biopsy. I had the most wonderful team in the room. They were all very compassionate and caring which helped me to stay calm.

The technician prepared me for the procedure which also involved some local anaesthetic to two points in my right breast and one in my left. To collect the specimen, the Core biopsy needle is inserted into the breast using ultrasound and when the technician believes they are at the correct site, feeling the breast to gain the correct position, they capture the sample by firing the needle into the mass. The hollow needle collects the sample and it is drawn out safely. I didn't feel any pain but heard a loud click and some pressure inside my breast, after each specimen capture. I did develop quite a few bruises and had some tenderness at the sites for a few days following the procedure, which was normal. After the procedure was finished, I was asked to stay in the waiting room. During this time, a lovely volunteer lady brought cups of tea to myself and the other ladies who were waiting. Thank god for volunteers!

During the wait time, I knew they were looking at the results of the ultrasound and determining whether they liked what they saw. After about an hour wait, the technician came and took me back to the room I had just been in. The doctor that was present came and explained to me that they would like to do another kind of biopsy, called a Stereotactic breast biopsy. She said this type of biopsy would give them a more accurate sample of tissue. The technician needed more information about a mass in my left breast as the ultrasound had not shown it clearly enough.

"Ok," I said, "Let's do it, I would rather have it done today than come back again." As they had the time as well, I wasn't going to pass that up.

A Stereotactic breast biopsy is a specific kind of biopsy. Radiologists use specialized mammography machines to help them pinpoint any suspicious areas. These machines provide radiologists with X-rays taken from two different angles. In a stereotactic breast biopsy, radiologists use two sets of images to guide them. Radiologists use the two sets of images to guide them to the area of concern and remove tissue samples. The samples are then analyzed to see if cancer is present.

I was shown into a room where a weird looking contraption was placed. It looked like an apparatus best suited to a gymnasium! I was asked to climb up a series of steps and then lay down on a table that had holes in it for your breasts to drop into. I feel they should make massage tables like this, as it would be a lot comfier!

Once I was on the table, lying on my stomach, the technician helped me get my breast into position, through the hole provided. I then had to turn my head in the other direction and stay as still as I could. It was not very comfortable at all. I didn't like laying on my stomach normally, so this was a bit hard to take. I stayed in this position for about thirty to fourty minutes.

The technician held my left breast in position while the other technician remotely moved the clamp for the breast into position. I was then left alone as the technician had gone behind the wall to look at the screens with her colleague. Once they had found the positions they wanted to sample, by moving the biopsy needle, the technicians would tell me they were about to take the core samples and again there was a loud clicking noise followed by slight pressure inside the breast, after each sample was taken. When the technicians had collected a few samples they inserted a small metal marker to show the position that the core samples had been taken from, in case of later possible surgery.

Once again, I cannot speak highly enough of the care and attention given to me during this rather trying day. All the staff were very respectful and showed compassion along with expertise. I knew I was in good hands.

After the procedure was finished, I was asked to get dressed and go to the Breast Clinic desk. I was given another appointment date for Wednesday 12th June 2013. We would be meeting with the doctor and discussing what type of surgery was needed, what treatment was needed and also talk about the reconstruction of the breast.

I had told Martin that if I needed a mastectomy for the right breast, I also wanted the other breast removed as well. I felt that if cancer could occur in the right breast, it could just as easily occur in the left breast. I didn't want to have to go through this journey again. Once was surely enough. My decision was based on how I felt and how I wanted to live my life, it was purely personal. Martin said he would support me in any choices that I made.

Martin came with me for the following Wednesday appointment. I really wanted him with me for support. He has always been my rock. I knew that he wanted to be there as well, no question. We went through the arrival process again at the Breast Clinic. Once my name was called, we again followed the doctor into the clinic room. I was told that the right breast did not have any further signs of cancer. The left breast results had not shown any cancer, only calcifications which are quite common. That was good news to me.

I asked Dr Kamyab what this meant for me and she looked at me and told me I would need a mastectomy of the right breast. I looked straight over at Martin.

"Yes that's what we thought, we were right," we said in unison.

I turned back to face Dr Kamyab and I can still to this day remember the look of compassion and empathy on her face. I was struck by this. I looked back at Martin and again towards my doctor and I gently patted her forearm.

"It's not your fault!" I told her.

I felt for Dr Kamyab and her position. As a doctor, she would have given this news to many other people in our position. I knew within my heart by this show of emotion, that my doctor cared about my welfare. I trusted that she would do all she could to help me.

Dr Kamyab told me that I would possibly also need chemotherapy along with the mastectomy. I looked straight at Martin as he knew I didn't really want chemo. I freaked out a little then, as I had seen my stepfather Jack when he was fighting lung cancer, suffer the effects of chemotherapy and I didn't want to suffer as he did. He had been given a diagnosis of three to six months and during those months had severe weight loss, no energy and no appetite. Dr Kamyab and the breast care nurse calmed me down by discussing the difference when having chemotherapy as a terminally ill patient and having it when your health is not as compromised. This talk helped me and gave me more understanding. I knew it was going to help my body combat any other cancer cells which may have gone unnoticed.

Dr Kamyab also discussed with me whether or not to have an Axillary clearance. She asked me if I would like to be part of a trial that was running in the breast clinic, but I declined. I was then told that she would perform an axillary clearance and the lymph nodes removed would be tested to see if they contained any cancer cells. I thought this was a good idea as it gave a more accurate picture of how far if at all, the cancer had spread.

Towards the end of the appointment, I asked Dr Kamyab about a prophylactic mastectomy of the left breast, as Martin and I had discussed. At the time I was undergoing my diagnosis,

Angelina Jolie was announcing to the world, her choice to have a double prophylactic mastectomy as she had the mutated BRCA 1 gene, which increased her risk of breast cancer developing. Every time we turned on the television there was always something about what was happening to her. We couldn't have tried to stop thinking about our diagnosis if we tried!

A prophylactic mastectomy is performed to reduce the risk of developing breast cancer, in one or both breasts.

When I told Dr Kamyab I wanted the second mastectomy, she said it should wait until we had undergone all our treatment for the right breast cancer. At first, in my confusion, I thought she was telling me I couldn't have it done at all, and I started to panic. I wanted to do everything I could to help myself and I didn't want someone telling me I couldn't do something. For me, this choice meant lessening my chances of having cancer develop in the left breast. The breast care nurse in the room looked at me.

"You can have it done, but the doctor is saying first deal with the breast cancer," she calmly said.

Dr Kamyab then said that after about twelve months, I could return to the breast centre and discuss having the prophylactic mastectomy. I was very happy to hear this news and I think Martin was as well.

Dr Kamyab looked through her appointment book and found a date of Friday 21st June 2013 and asked us if that date would be okay to have the surgery. Martin and I were both surprised but really happy that it was going to happen so quickly, and agreed straight away. I had to fill out some paperwork for the operation, which had all my personal information on it as well as a detailed description of what the operation was about and what was going to be done. After the doctor filled out all her parts, I then read it and signed the forms.

There is a constant Q & A during any pre-admission and surgery to make sure you know what is going to be done and to check that you are the person listed on the paperwork. I was always happy to answer the questions as I knew the nurses and doctors were doing their best to ensure everything went smoothly for every patient.

After a few calls were made, we were fitted in for an appointment in the Pre Admission clinic at one pm that day. We thanked Dr Kamyab and said we looked forward to seeing her on the 21st June.

While we were waiting for the appointment Martin and I went downstairs to one of the cafes for some lunch. After we ordered, we sat looking at each other in a state of shock. After so many weeks of waiting and testing and more waiting, everything suddenly seemed real. I was going to have my breast removed to save my life.

Martin's perspective on Diagnosis

Reading through what Caroline has written in this chapter brought up a lot of emotion. To look back at this initial stage of our five-year journey turned me into a blubbering mess yet again. And as we go further into these memoirs I am sure there will be many more tears and giggles and terrible spelling and punctuation. I will do my best to put my perspective on what has happened, what we have been through and what we hope the future will bring for us.

Hearing someone you love so deeply being diagnosed with a life-threatening disease, is one shock that I don't think I will ever recover from. The original diagnosis in 2004 from the "wonky" pap smear was bad enough. To be facing a diagnosis of the big "C", is something that I am sure no one ever expects to happen to them. I am sure that is why, as mentioned previously, I proceeded to stick my head in the sand and pretend that everything was just dandy. I am sure there is some sort of psychological reason for this and from what I heard about my reaction, I think

I would have made the perfect case study. But even though I refused to admit that anything was happening, I am sure that I managed, through the fog, to be supportive of my beautiful wife. And to me, that is what my role was to be. I was to be a listener, carer when needed, driver, supporter and the person who would try to make her as comfortable as possible, whatever she was going through.

I couldn't understand what Caroline was feeling, as it wasn't happening to me. I would sit and listen to everything she had read and to be honest, I believe most of it went in one ear and out of the other. Not because I didn't want to listen or because I didn't understand what the bloody hell she was talking about, but because I didn't want to believe that this could be happening to us. I think that things became clear when we finally met with Doctor Kamyab. I sat and listened to what she said and I think this was the first time that I really understood what we were facing- and to be honest, that there was a light at the end of the tunnel.

As Caroline has mentioned, we had talked about possible treatments that may happen and we had pretty much decided that a mastectomy was going to be the initial treatment. So when we were told that mastectomy it is, it didn't really shock me, but confirmed that we were going to beat this thing. I know it was a bit early to be thinking like this, but obviously the time I had spent listening to Caroline talk about what she had researched, had really sunk in through the fog. In my mind, by removing the cancerous breast we removed the cancer. Maybe I under-thought this and made it a bit more simple than it really was, but it is what got me through.

I had started a new job on the 12th of May 2013. A week later, I was telling my new boss that we had received this news and I might need a day off here and there to attend appointments with my wife. My Manager and the company I worked for (and still do) were very supportive and I attended as many appointments as I could, but bearing in mind that I would probably need days off for possible treatments, I did miss some. This was hard to do but necessary as life still goes on around you.

Talking was a very important part of this process. Caroline and I talked and discussed everything. Our moods went up and down but we ALWAYS had each other to bounce off of. I remember a day when I was driving to Mandurah, feeling quite sad. Luckily, Caroline must have picked up on my mood and called. After the crying stopped (oh yes, I am not ashamed to admit that there was plenty of that) we, as usual, laughed. It was very rare that we both had a down moment together, but there were some and later in the book, you will hear about a particular one that we look back on and laugh now but at the time was the end of the world as we knew it.

As we move from diagnosis to treatment I wish to make some personal observations. I believe the following:

- There is no shame in showing your emotions.
- There is no shame in talking to someone professionally or to your mates.
- I wish I had believed this for a lot longer than I have.

I should have talked more to other people, as it may have helped me to shovel away the sand and see things more clearly. I was offered the chance to talk to someone by the excellent and very helpful people at Breast cancer Care WA - free of charge, numerous times, but in my infinite wisdom, declined. Please accept these offers, even if it's just to see if they help. You won't have to do it again if you don't feel it was for you. You won't even have to tell anyone you did it. You might be surprised. It might actually help.

Chapter 2

Treatment

At this stage, after the meeting with Dr. Kamyab, the only treatment we knew we needed was a mastectomy. It wouldn't be until after the operation and the post-op appointment, we would find out if there was any adjunct treatment needed.

Martin and I made our way to the pre-admission clinic after lunch, to get all the testing done in readiness for the upcoming operation on 21st June 2013. This clinic is for anyone having an operation, not purely for breast cancer patients.

If you need to visit this clinic my same suggestions apply as for the breast clinic. As the doctors are visiting during their work day, they are sometimes delayed. I learned from the first visit to the Breast clinic and from then on I was prepared. Take a snack, a book, a friend if at all possible, although I often liked to chat with the other patients waiting.

I remember one clinic I attended, after my second operation. In the waiting room were myself and two other ladies. I could hear one of the ladies, seated next to me, talking with her husband about what was going to be happening to her. She had breast cancer. After a few minutes of listening to her, she paused in her conversation. I can't remember exactly what I said to her that started our conversation, but within minutes we were discussing her diagnosis and I told her about my operations and treatment. Her husband was listening intently as well. We talked for a few minutes during which time another lady had come into the waiting room. The lady I had been speaking to was then called up and she and her husband left the room. The new lady who had walked into the waiting room caught my eye and said she couldn't help overhearing what myself and the previous lady had been discussing. She then started telling me about her diagnosis, again breast cancer, and once again my story was told. She asked me questions about different things and I tried to answer her with the knowledge

I had learned, but I also told her about the My Journey Kit and the BCNA website and also Breast Cancer Care W.A. A short while later this lady was also called in for her appointment. After she left the room, the lady who was seated across the room from me, and had been since I arrived, turned to look at me.

She said, "I've been listening to you talking to those ladies. I really feel you're going to help a lot more people in the future. You are such a kind and helpful person to tell them your story."

I was really touched by her words. I didn't think anything about telling my story. It was personal to me, but if my story could help alleviate someone else's shock and confusion and give them some hope and understanding then I would gladly tell it. I believe this is how the idea for this book came about. When I talked to people though, I always told them that the choices I made were done entirely from a personal viewpoint and they should research and make their decisions based on what their needs are. I have never told people what I thought they should or shouldn't do.

Martin and I entered the clinic waiting room where we were greeted by a lovely friendly man, who is the admissions clerk. He has been present at all of my clinic visits and it's nice to see his friendly smiling face. My name was taken and crossed off his list and he let us know that as we were an add-on, the wait could be a little while. Today we would be seeing a nurse and an anaesthetist. Normally we would also see a doctor that is attached to the breast clinic but as we had just seen Dr. Kamyab we wouldn't be seeing a doctor that day. We thanked him and took our seats.

After an hour or so wait, I was called by a nurse, who firstly weighed me, then measured my height and then took me to a clinic room. Here she went through all the paperwork and discussed with me what the operation involved. As I was having a mastectomy, the entire breast was going to be removed including the nipple and as much tissue and skin as was deemed necessary to give a good clear margin, which is where no cancer cells were present. Sometimes depending on the stage and size of the cancer present, there can be nipple sparing and also skin sparing of the breast. In Angelina Jolie's case, she had skin and nipple sparing, prophylactic double mastectomy, as cancer was not yet present in her breasts.

Dr. Kamyab had told me at our earlier meeting that she would perform an Axillary Clearance.

During our meeting she had also asked me if I would like to join a clinical trial for a new medication, which was hoped would reduce the size of cancer tumours before surgery. Martin and I declined. I was happy though that I would have the axillary clearance. To me, it represented another way to make sure there was no cancer left behind. In my case, however, it did come with its own after effects! More on this in Chapter four.

I asked the nurse how long I would be in the hospital for and she said if the operation went according to plan, I would only be in overnight. What! I couldn't believe it would be such a short time. That was quite a shock. She said there would be some drainage tubes attached to me that I would go home with and that the hospital would arrange for Silver Chain to visit me at home.

Silver Chain are an amazing organisation. Part of the service they offer involve nurses who are able to visit patients in their homes and give them medical attention, so the patient doesn't have to take up a much-needed hospital bed.

The nurse continued to ask me questions about my health and about medications I was taking for

Rheumatoid arthritis. I was diagnosed with this chronic disease in December 2012. She then took some blood samples, I'm O negative. I was asked if I had any other questions.

"Yeh millions," I replied with a smile on my face.

The nurse gave me a tube of antiseptic body wash to use on the morning of the operation and a brochure about the upcoming operation for me to read. I then went back to the waiting room and gave Martin a detailed description of what had occurred.

After a short while, the anaesthetist called me and I followed him into another room. He checked again that all the details on the paperwork were correct. We discussed the operation and what it entailed. He then made me move my neck around and up and down and poke out my tongue. He said he was doing these checks to ensure he wouldn't have any issues when intubating me (putting a tube down my throat) for the operation. I had only undergone two previous surgeries in the past for a tubal ligation and cone biopsy for the CIN 1 result, which had both been problem free, so he was hoping for the same result. The anaesthetist asked me if I had any other questions but as I hadn't, he said goodbye and I made my way back out to my anxiously waiting hubby.

We were told we could go home then, with instructions on how to get to the Day surgery ward for the 21st June and also that a nurse would call us the night before, to let us know what time to get to the hospital. As the surgery list is only prepared the night before, you don't know whether the surgery will be performed in the morning or the afternoon. We thanked the clerk and made our way out to the car.

On the way home, we were both in our own little worlds, trying to process everything we had just been told. I was really happy that the operation was going to be so soon. I just wanted the breast and cancer off my body. I hadn't really given much thought to after the operation. At this point, all I could think about was surviving and that meant getting rid of the problem. I had seen a picture in one of the booklets that came with the My Journey kit, of a lady that had a mastectomy. The photograph was taken a while after the operation. I know this now, as when I had my mastectomy, it took about a year before my scar looked as faded as the picture.

As we now had some definite dates I called my

manager at work to let him know. Dr. Kamyab had suggested I have two weeks off work and I also couldn't drive for two weeks. He was so understanding and very supportive. I let him know that I couldn't tell him of any further treatment required until after the operation and the post-op appointment, which had been made for the 3rd of July. Martin had also let his boss know and so he was given the Friday of the operation off. I had said that I thought I would be fine at home from the Monday onwards, as it would really just be rest and recuperation.

As I now knew what initial treatment I would need, I called Breast Cancer Care W.A and asked to speak to someone as I had quite a few questions. I was told that a McGrath breast care nurse would call me back later that day.

In the late afternoon, I received a call from Moira, who became my Florence Nightingale. I can often go off on tangents when I'm having a conversation, and if you speak to those that know me they'll all agree. It can be a bit challenging sometimes keeping up with me!! Moira handled me with no problems. I asked all sorts of questions regarding the upcoming mastectomy. What would happen, before and after?

Moira had such a calming effect on me and answered all my questions with honesty. Even now when I think of her, I feel a sort of calmness. After every phone call, I would feel a sense of positivity. I'm sure people got tired of hearing her name but for me, Moira offered a certain kind of support that I really needed.

It was also lucky for me as Moira had been a breast care nurse at SCGH and so she already knew the doctors, nurses and physiotherapists who worked there. This helped me a lot as well, as I now had first-hand knowledge which gave me a sense of security. Moira encouraged me to ask questions and slowed me down when I jumped the gun, in regard to things that would happen in the future.

Every week I got a call from Moira. From before my first operation until after my later treatments. I looked forward to that call immensely and I even wrote things down when they came to me during the week. The Breast Care nurses that work with Breast Cancer Care W.A. are funded purely by public donations and fundraising. If you would ever like to donate to a worthy cause, this one is one of the best. At the end of my chemo treatment, I wanted to thank

Moira somehow. So, I arranged a morning tea with the girls at BCCWA to surprise Moira. I went in to the offices at the end of the week with flowers and a cake (see below). It was so lovely to meet face-to-face, the face behind the voice that had calmed me, taught me and guided me over the worst months of my life. Thank you again Moira and BCCWA.

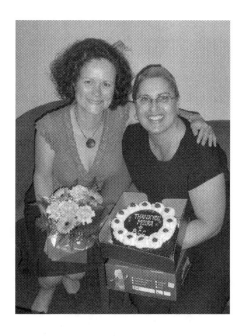

For the next two weeks, I researched topics that interested me. I primarily used the books that I had received from the My Journey Kit, also The BCNA website, Breast Cancer Care W.A website and the Cancer Council W.A. website. By doing my bit of research, I felt I had some semblance of control over what might happen to me. I would listen to the doctor's recommendations, but I also wanted to feel in charge of what might happen to my body.

I had started to research the type of breast reconstructions that were available after having a mastectomy. I would discuss these with Martin and I would tell him my reasons for wanting/not wanting certain choices. As some of these choices depend on the type of treatment plan needed, I couldn't make a final decision until after the mastectomy. I will offer more information on these in the next chapter on Reconstruction.

During this time, I also chatted a lot to my wonderful work colleague Peng. She helped me more than she knows and for this love and support, I will always treasure her friendship. I was able to discuss anything with her and she took it all in her stride, even when it may have been confrontational. I was very thankful to be able to continue work and having her friendship and listening ear, especially from the female perspective, supported me wonderfully. We laughed often during this trying time, and it was a blessing to be able to go to work and forget about things for a few hours a day if I wanted to or to chew her ear off as I did quite a bit. I'm sure Peng would agree with me there.

I will share something with you now that is quite personal, but Martin and I want to increase the readers' awareness of how a cancer diagnosis can affect every part of your life.

The date of the operation was fast approaching. As a sort of last HURRAH!! and goodbye to one of my two, I won't say normal, breasts, we decided to go to the Hyatt Hotel for the weekend and have a little bit of fun, I hope you know what I mean!

Well, let's just say that there wasn't much fun, as there were too many tears. We both took turns crying, then we'd switch to having a laugh, then we'd go back to crying. Put it this way and word to the wise, if I had the chance again, I would not spend the money at a hotel, I'd stay at home in my nice cheap comfy bed.

I believe I was sad not for the fact that I would lose a breast, as I knew I would eventually gain another one, but as for a time, I would only have one breast. I didn't know how that was going to affect my own self-esteem. How would I see myself? I was hoping that my wonderful husband would still find me attractive. Would he still want me even though I only had one breast? I felt as though one thing was happening which was positive, but it may cause other things to happen that may be a struggle. I'll tell you more about the after-effects of surgery later.

On the evening of the 20th of June, the night before the operation, a nurse from SCGH called me at home. She asked me to be at the hospital at six thirty am, as I would be having my surgery just after lunch. She also asked me to remember to fast from ten pm that night, with only a small sip of water in the morning, to wash with the antiseptic body wash I was given at the Pre-admission visit, and also to not use any deodorant or moisturiser.

The next morning, we headed to the hospital and booked in at about six forty-five am. There are many people having day surgery so my advice is to be patient. We were called up to the desk and offered our Medicare card and the clerk checked all my personal information was correct. She then gave me a yellow envelope which contained the paperwork for the operation and asked us to make our way upstairs to the Day Surgery Ward.

When we arrived upstairs I handed the

envelope to the clerk there and we were asked to take a seat and wait for a nurse to call my name. While we waited Martin and I both read a book we'd bought with us. I'd prefer to read rather than stare aimlessly around, I think it also helped to calm my nerves. I made sure I had worn comfy warm clothes as I didn't know how long the wait would be. It can get a bit chilly sitting around waiting so remember to dress warmly and comfortably.

After about two hours a nurse called my name and asked me to change into one of their lovely blue gowns. To enhance the beauty of the gown, I also had a gorgeous pair of paper bikini bottoms, which I cheekily tied up very nicely at the sides. Ohhh I looked good! Not. I rang the bell after changing and the nurse came and got me and I followed her into the ward.

In the ward, patients were waiting in various stages of readiness for their operations. Remember that any staff member that comes to prepare you for anything to do with your operation, and there may be three to four different people, will ask you the same set of questions. Don't get mad, as this is a requirement to ensure the right person is having the right operation. Would you like to wake up with a missing breast if you should have had a knee reconstruction?

The male nurse started off by tucking me up into a nice comfy bed with those wonderful cotton blankets that are so warm. Martin settled in next to me on a chair. I could feel him starting to worry. Then it was question time from the nurse. Who am I? Where do I live? Address?, What operation am I having done today?, Any allergies? Etc. etc. I was then measured for compression stockings. These are worn before, during and after an operation, to assist with blood circulation and prevent blood clots when lying prone for any amount of time. The nurse went and got the right size and helped me put them on. I loved these, they were so comfortable and warm. After the nurse had finished we were left alone for a while.

I can't say I was scared while I waited to be taken for the operation, maybe a bit nervous. I was just so ready to do this. This was my life and if this operation was what had to happen for me to survive, then so be it. Martin and I looked at each other a lot, held hands and shared a few kisses. He had decided as the operation was going to take about two hours that he would go into Subiaco on the bus and have some lunch, as he hadn't eaten either, in support of me. We were told that after the operation it might be a couple of hours before I was ready to see him. I told him to go home and I'd see him in the morning.

He kept saying to me "I'm not going home today until I've seen you and I know you're all right. I don't care what time it is."

The next person to appear was the anaesthetist, a different one from the one I had met at the Pre Admission clinic. You may find that you see a few different doctors for any one scenario, as they may be a part of the same team. The same questions as before were asked of me and I was also asked to move my head about and poke out my tongue.

Finally, at around two thirty pm, the orderlies came and got me ready to take to the operating theatre. Martin and I shared a big kiss or two and he was told that the operation would take about one and a half to two hours. After that time he could call the day surgery ward to find out how everything had gone. I was then wheeled away. Being wheeled through the back corridors of the hospital was quite weird. You get to see things that are otherwise kept from public eyes.

I was parked in the waiting room of the operating theatre and a nurse came to insert a cannula into my arm. This is what the anaesthetist would use to administer the anaesthetic. I chatted with her for a few minutes and was then wheeled into theatre. I then had to try and manoeuver onto a really thin, cold operating table, the staff were very helpful though. My body got cold pretty quickly, so a nurse got a heated blanket and put that over me, which was nice as it made me feel safe. Dr. Kamyab arrived and said hello to me and asked how I was. I told her I was ready to go. The anaesthetist put a mask over my mouth and nose and asked me to take a few deep breaths in and out. I started to lose consciousness quite quickly and was then out for the count.

I will now include an excerpt from my journal which I wrote a few days later; *"Upon coming out of anaesthetic OMG!!!! Pain. Asked for pain relief and then not too bad. Had op at 3.15pm. In Day Ward at 7 pm. Sleepy"*.

I was told by the anaesthetist at my pre-admission meeting to remember to take some nice deep breaths after having surgery, as it would help my lungs get back to normal quicker. As I'm a stickler for the rules, I stupidly took deep breaths right after waking up. Idiot! No wonder it was painful. Once I used my foggy brain and thought about it, I took shallower breaths. Please learn from my stupidity.

After the operation, while in the recovery ward a nurse told me that it had all gone well. It had taken longer than first thought, about two and a half hours. She said I would be moved to the Day Surgery Ward as soon as my obs were stable. Every thirty minutes after my operation, my blood pressure and temperature were taken. I was attached to an I.V. also, as I was being given intravenous antibiotics to guard against infection. I was aware at some stage of a feeling as though someone was squeezing my calf muscles.

"Who is squeezing my legs?" I slowly asked the nurse in my drug-induced voice.

She told me it was the compression cuffs around my calves. This device is used to help in the prevention of blood clots by assisting blood flow. The cuff fills with air and squeezes the calf muscle and then goes down. They are helpful when the patient can't move around. I found them comfortable and soothing.

I started to get an itchy face as well, and so the lovely post-op nurse wiped my face with a warm face cloth. She told me it was probably a little irritated by the antiseptic wash that was wiped over parts of my body before the operation. Such wonderful care and attention. A small gesture such as having my face gently wiped, made me feel better. I have a profound respect for our nurses and the amazing work they do in caring for us, when we are ill and at our most vulnerable.

I also had two drains in the chest area on the right-hand side. One situated under where the breast had curved against the skin and another slightly around the side of the breast. These drains had a couple of stitches holding them in and were coiled around inside the chest wall to ensure the wound drained and a haematoma (swelling) did not develop. The drainage tube was attached to clear plastic bottles with measurements up the side. The nurses would be able to measure the amount of liquid being drained. These bottles were housed in pretty little shoulder bags made from colourful cotton material. These bags are made by volunteers at the hospital. It makes getting around with drainage bottles much easier that's for sure. A big Thankyou to the lovely volunteers at S.C.G.H for making these bags, as I have used many sets of them throughout the years.

After a couple of hours of half-hourly, then hourly obs, I was wheeled into the Day Surgery ward where I would be spending the night. This ward is a mix of men and women and is quite a big room with rows of beds, not individual rooms. I was parked in my space and made comfortable by the orderlies and went back to sleep.

My poor worried husband popped his head around the curtains of my cubicle around seven fifteen pm, after being told he could finally come to see me. He had been sitting in the waiting room all on his own after coming back from having lunch around five pm. I was, needless to say, still quite groggy, so after a quick kiss and trying to let him know I was alright, he took himself off home to bed. He told me he would return in the morning to take me home. At that stage, the thought of home was far from my mind.

I slept fitfully for the first couple of hours, as the nurses were still doing hourly obs. I also didn't take my earplugs, which I sleep with at night, so it was a little bit weird hearing the nightly noises from the ward. About one am the nurse came to give me an injection of Heparin which injected into my stomach. It's fifty/fifty whether you get the after-burn or not. It's like being stung by a bee. This injection was an anticoagulant (blood thinning) medication. Then there was finally the trip to the bathroom.

So picture this. It's the middle of the night. I buzz the lovely night nurse and say I need to go to the bathroom. I still to this day cannot use bedpans. How can I pee in a pan in bed, when my hoo-ha is up in the air above my pelvis and not under it like it usually is? The nurse was then forced to get a shower commode chair for transport.

So, the first step, the nurse has to take off the massage cuffs which are velcroed on to the lower part of my legs. Secondly, the nurse has to bring the IV drip stand around to the same side of the bed that I'm trying to get out of. Thirdly, I carefully sit on the side of the bed for a while to let the blood slowly get to my head and to wait for some nausea to pass. And so on. Trying to get myself up off the bed was the hardest, as I had to hook the drainage bag over my other shoulder being careful not to pull at it while trying not to pull the IV drip from my other arm and all the while trying to place myself over the bottomless chair!! Obviously with a lot of help. As the nurse pushes me on the chair towards the bathroom, I'm pushing the IV stand as well, with my bare bottom hanging out the bottom of a bottomless toilet chair! What a sight that would have been? The commode shower chair allows you to be wheeled over a toilet and do what you need to do, without getting out of the chair itself. While trying to go to the bathroom, I have an almighty heave-ho from the stomach, classily pre-empted by the nurse, who had already handed me a little bag to catch the contents, but then feel better for it. So it's then back to bed in reverse order, and then to two hourly obs till morning.

My journal entry suggested I didn't get much sleep that night. *"Soooo tired. Not much sleep at all. Needle in stomach at 1 am. Arm stiff. Drains in. Drip up. Electric massagers on (like these a lot). Fun going to the loo."*

Some time after the nurse put me back to bed, she came to see the lady that was in the bed next to mine. As she left the cubicle, I heard the nurse ask the lady if she would like a cup of tea and a biscuit. Well, I was certainly going to get in on this action, so I quietly spoke up.

"Could I have a cup of tea too please?" I asked in my sweetest voice.

"You sure can," answered the nurse, "Biscuit as well?"

"Yes please," I answered, not believing my good luck.

My lovely nurse Liz, soon returned with manna from heaven. A hot sweet cup of tea and a couple of biscuits. When I think of that now, it still makes me feel good! Talk about bedside manner. I was lucky enough to be cared for by Liz, for two future operations.

The following morning Martin arrived about eight thirty am and it was lovely to see him and have a hug. I wasn't in any pain, I was well supplied with pain relief, just a little tired and shell-shocked I think. I knew I certainly didn't want to look at my chest and I tried not to look down. I had been a size 14D so there was a sizable difference now, in how my chest looked underneath my pyjama top. Remember to buy a top that buttons up at the front, as it's much easier to have anything seen to when you can just undo the buttons and not have to try to take a top off over your head.

I hadn't wanted Martin to see my chest, so I had asked the nurse earlier in the morning if she could help me to put on the PJ top. When he arrived, he helped me into my comfy trousers and we waited for the medical team to arrive so we could go home.

Around ten am, I was visited by a physiotherapist from the breast centre, who gave me a couple of exercises to do. I found I was able to do them gently straight away which surprised me. When I went home I did them religiously. The exercise involved gently lifting my right elbow forwards and upwards towards the ceiling and also then out to the side.

I was also seen by the team of doctors that were on call that day. They checked the wound site and the drainage amounts that the nurse had collected overnight. They were happy with the results. We were given our first post-op appointment date for 3rd July 2013. I was told that a Silver Chain nurse would be coming to visit me at home every day to check the fluid outputs of the drains. When they were at an acceptable level of fluid drainage, which was around fifty ml, the drains would be removed. By this stage, I was really tired and just wanted to go home. The nurse called an orderly who arrived with a wheelchair and together with my hubby, wheeled me to the front doors.

During my stay at the hospital, I received a Zonta breast care cushion. I can't recall whether it was a nurse or the physiotherapist that gave it to me. These cushions are again made by wonderful volunteers from Zonta clubs around Australia, who hold sewing bees to create these lovely cushions. The cushions are then donated for men and women who are recovering from breast surgery. Zonta club members help women around the world to empower themselves, by delivering projects both locally and internationally and providing educational opportunities and advocating to improve women's lives.

My trip home in the car was made more comfortable by using this soft silky cushion. I placed it underneath my right arm and it created a lovely cushion between my chest wall and my arm. This simple item brought a world of comfort to me over the next few weeks. I also used it whenever I went out in the car and also when walking around. The cushion helped me to adjust to the missing breast, by supplying a form and allowed me to have my right arm down by my side, without feeling that something was not quite right.

During the ride home, Martin and I just chilled and listened to the radio. I really wanted to sleep and it was so nice to be out of the hospital and to know I was going home. It was amazing to feel the sun on my face and look at the scenery on the way home. My gorgeous hubby was so attentive to my needs and was trying to miss all the bumps in the road. Quite a feat when you live in the Perth hills. After a one hour journey, we finally made it. Martin helped me inside and into my waiting bed, plumped up with soft pillows and it was such a beautiful feeling to know I was now home. This is from my journal: *"Home, ah. Sleep in my lovely bed with my lovely family around me. Slept for four hours in the afternoon. Had a good night's sleep with my hubby next to me."*

When I was settled in bed, Martin asked the children if they wanted to come in and see me which of course they did. They were both very tentative and hugged me carefully. Of course, weepy old me starts crying, as I was so glad to be home. They asked how I was feeling and I told them I wasn't in any pain and I was really happy to be home. I think they were too. I don't think it matters sometimes what capacity a mother has, as long as she is in the family home.

I don't know about other couples, but I have found that Martin and I like a particular side of the bed to sleep on. I usually got out of bed on my left-hand side. As my right breast had been removed, and I had two drains attached to the bottles in the little bag, we had decided that we would switch sides of the bed until the drains were removed. I tell you it made getting up for the toilet at night much easier. Thank you, babe! I was able to get out of the bed easily by swinging my legs out first, then picking up the bag and hanging it on my shoulder and then getting up and walking to the bathroom. Once there, I put the bag on the floor, did my business, and put the bag once again on my shoulder. Sometimes if I wasn't thinking, I'd go to get out of bed and forget to take the bag with me and it was only when I felt a little pull that I'd remember and pick it up.

As we're talking about the bathroom, I will mention one fact that I feel very strongly about. As I had had powerful drugs to put me to sleep for the operation, and some strong pain medication (Endone and Panamax) for the first few days after, I became very constipated - a matter which I had never suffered with. It took about 3-4 doses of Metamucil and a couple of days for everything to go back to normal. I learned from this incident and so two days before every future operation, I made sure I started taking Metamucil twice daily. I never had a problem after that, so please consider this little helpful hint or pass it on.

By late afternoon on Saturday, I was feeling like I needed something stronger than Panadol so I took one of the Endone tablets. It was such a weird feeling taking this medication, as I had never taken anything stronger than a Panadol before. Within a few minutes, I felt a slowness and depth in my breathing, and everything seemed to go in slow motion. The pain disappeared which was really good, however, I didn't like the slowness of my breathing. I didn't take another Endone after the first one, I didn't really like the effects and I was lucky enough that Panamax did a good pain relief job if I took them every six hours. I also drank plenty of water which helped to flush my kidneys and any residual medication from the operation.

On Sunday after the operation, the Silver Chain nurse made her first visit to the house. She measured the liquid in both of the drains and marked the amount on the side of the bottle with a permanent marker. The amounts were written in a folder that I had been given, so the next nurse could follow along from there. The nurse wasn't sure if she would be seeing me again the next day or whether it would be someone else. There was quite a lot of liquid in the bottles, one, in particular, had one hundred and forty mills that had drained out since having the operation the day before. This shows the importance of having the drains put in, otherwise, a haematoma could develop. As the liquid output was still high, the nurse said the drains would stay in. This was fine with me as they were not too bothersome.

A journal entry from the day: *"Getting around much easier. Sore back. Doing arm exercises every hour or so. My beautiful sissy bought up so much lovely food. Mummy came with her to organise the week with my baby. I wouldn't have done half as well if I didn't have the loving care from my gorgeous hubby. He's my rock, more than he knows. I'm a very lucky lady. Love ya babe xx. Aunty Jules lasagne OMG!!"*

In the My Journey booklet, on the Journal entry pages, there is a space to write the date and also a space to circle from number one to number five, to show how you are feeling on that day. For the Friday night after the operation, I had later circled a number three, which was average. On Saturday morning, I had circled a number one, which was very poor. You have read about that difficult night. By the Sunday morning, I was circling number four, which meant I was feeling good!

To help my recovery, I would get up at some stage of the day and gently walk around the house. My mum's long-term best friend who we referred to as Aunty Gerry, had brought me the softest cuddliest blanket after the operation, which was quite large. As the tubing and the bottles were quite confrontational for the children to see, when I walked around the house I would drape the blanket over my body and the bottle bag, which successfully covered everything. In that way, we continued on quite normally which was good for all of us. Thank you again, Aunty Gerry, I do still love that blanket.

Martin went back to work on the Monday morning and left me with strict instructions. Don't do this, don't do that, don't look here and don't look there! Ladies, I'm sure you know how it is when you're not in charge of running your household. We do things the way we like them done. But as I slowly walked around the house once everyone had gone for the day, I was so deeply appreciative and thankful that I had met and married an amazing man, who looked after me so well. The house was nice and tidy, dishes were done and even the washing was done. All I had to concentrate on was getting better. I was able to carefully get my own breakfast, which also helped me to feel better and not so dependent on everyone.

Around mid-morning, a Silver Chain nurse came again to check the fluid levels in the drain bottles. At last one of them was under the required minimum level and could be taken out. The nurse moved a button on top of the drainage bottle to the off position, so that there was no longer any suction coming from the bottle. I didn't know what to expect, so I just followed the instructions of the nurse. Firstly, she had to remove all the sticky adhesive dressings from over the top of the tubing. Then she had to snip the little stitch that was keeping the drainage tube in place, against my chest wall. Then while I was lying half on my side, I took a slow deep breath in, and the nurse gently pulled the drain out from my body in a smooth fluid motion. Done! The nurse popped a small dressing over the wound, completed her paperwork and went off to her next patient. I had a two-hour sleep.

Later in the afternoon, my mum came for a

visit. She was sitting on the end of my bed and we were talking about how I felt and she asked if anything needed to be done. While we were chatting, I kept feeling as though I had a wet patch on my pyjama shirt. Mum and I finally had a closer look and we found that the dressing the nurse had put on earlier, had not adhered properly and the drain wound was leaking a little fluid. Mum to the rescue! My lovely, caring mum had previously worked as a Care Aid for Silver Chain, so she got to work.

We found my container that held all our medicines and plasters and she cut and measured what she thought we would need. As I have mentioned previously, I did not want to see the surgery scar or look at the place where my breast used to be, but as this leak had occurred, mum and I now had to see it. We went into the bathroom together and mum helped me take off my PJ top.

It was a huge shock to see the large gap where my breast used to sit. Very confrontational for me and also for mum. We both got quite teary. I was a little bit bruised and could really see how much tissue had been removed. My chest wall looked a little concave. I remembered Dr. Kamyab had wanted to have a very clear margin in order to get all the cancerous tissue the first time. I could just see the scar as a dark line underneath the bandages. There really wasn't much to it at all. Considering the size and quantity of tissue that was removed, the scar was only about six centimetres long and Dr. Kamyab had made it in the shape of an arch. She later said this was so I could wear a plunging neckline and no scar would show. What a lovely doctor to be thinking of the outcome for me, in the way of making the scar look as good as it could be.

So once the initial shock was over, mum got to work. I went back and laid on the bed and she got the plasters she needed and stuck me back together again. This called for the best remedy in the world, a nice hot cup of tea. Thanks, mum!!

I had decided that since I had seen the scar, I might as well let Martin see it as well, when he got home from work that day. It needed to happen sooner or later. I hadn't shown him anything at all, at that stage. He could obviously see through my PJ top that I only had one breast, but this was different. I explained what had happened that day and how mum had looked after me and what I had decided. As he sat on the end of the bed, I unbuttoned my top to show him the result of the surgery. I was really uncertain as to what his reaction would be. He got quite emotional and teary and then he gently kissed my surgery scar. He said he was sad and teary for me, as I was the one that had to go through it. He was just happy that he still had me. He said those words to me many times over the next few years. God, I love this man. After this experience, we didn't look back.

The second drain was removed two days later. A wonderful day. I no longer needed to carry around the drain bags and worry about the tubes. I was feeling quite good, even though I still had a little pain and discomfort and was a bit stiff. I was doing my arm exercises every day but was feeling a tightness up the inside of my right arm from the armpit to past the elbow. Martin and I weren't quite sure what was causing the pain but as we had the post-op appointment coming up in a few days, we knew we could check with someone then. Until that time, I continued to take Panadol and gently increased my time spent walking around the house and garden.

During the two weeks that I was recovering at home until the post-op appointment, I had read about treatments that are used as an adjunct to surgery. Treatments such as chemotherapy and radiation are quite common ones. As I had already decided that I wanted breast reconstruction using implants, I had read that as the breast skin can be affected after radiation treatment, the skin can sometimes be too thin for implants. In regard to chemotherapy, I had seen my stepfather Jack suffer the effects when he was diagnosed with Lung cancer. He was told by his doctors that he may have three months to live without the chemo or six months with it, so of course, he opted for the six-month treatment option. As he was battling a terminal diagnosis and his body was already struggling, the treatment left him debilitated. Whenever I thought of having chemotherapy as my treatment, my mind always flashed back to poor Jack and I knew I didn't want to suffer as he had. Martin and I had talked about treatment options and I was sure that I didn't want chemo.

On the 3rd July 2013, Martin and I attended the post operation appointment (post-op) at the Breast Clinic. I was very hesitant about this visit as Dr. Kamyab would be telling us how the operation had gone, whether the lymph nodes under my right armpit contained any cancer cells and also if there was any other treatment required. Martin had told his boss that he wanted to attend the appointment with me to support me and once again his boss readily agreed. This was a new job that Martin had started only weeks before my diagnosis. The company did and continued to do all they could to ensure Martin didn't miss any important appointments.

We went through the check-in procedure at the clinic and didn't have to wait long before Dr. Kamyab called us in. My heart was in my mouth, I was so nervous about the results. We sat down and as always a lovely breast care nurse was also present. Dr. Kamyab started off by saying that the operation was successful and that a clear margin had been gained. The results of the axillary clearance were very good, as zero out of seventeen nodes taken were positive for any cancer cells. I was really relieved to hear this and by the tears that had started to flow down Martin's face, he was too! This was good news at last.

As to any further treatment required, Dr. Kamyab started off by saying that chemotherapy would be a good option for me to destroy any other cancer cells which may be present in my body. As soon as she said this I started to freak out a bit. I looked over at Martin and I knew he could tell what I was thinking. I told Dr. Kamyab that I had seen my stepdad suffer the effects of chemo while going through treatment for lung cancer and I didn't want to suffer as he did. I was sitting there picturing my children and my mum seeing me suffering as Jack had, God I didn't want them to go through that. After a few minutes, Dr. Kamyab and the breast care nurse explained to me that when a body is already being ravaged by disease, sometimes the effects of chemotherapy can seem worse, as it puts an already stressed body under more stress. In my situation, however, as my body was not under such physical stress, the effects of chemotherapy may not be as drastic. As the doctor was talking, I was thinking about the things she was saying and could see her point of view quite clearly. I felt quite strong and positive in myself, so after a brief discussion, I readily agreed to this treatment.

Dr. Kamyab also said I would be required to have some radiation treatment. My smile turned down at that. I had seen the after effects on the skin from radiation treatment when my dad had uvula cancer. I again looked at Martin. I don't think he knew what to do or say. He knew how I felt about both treatments but he wanted me to survive, as much as I did. I tried not to let the news get me down and so I let Dr. Kamyab continue. She said I would also need to have some hormone therapy. I would be seeing an Oncologist to discuss the chemotherapy and hormone treatment and also a Radiation Oncologist for the radiation treatment. We were told we had an appointment that day with the Radiation Oncologist. Well, that was a lot to take in. I was told that in another week I could take off the steri strips from the surgery scar. We said a big thank you to Dr. Kamyab, who said she would probably see me in a year or so to discuss the breast reconstruction surgery.

After leaving the office, one of the breast care nurses asked me my bra size. The wonderful company Berlei, offers women who have had breast surgery a My Care Kit free of charge. Each My Care Kit includes a DVD called Strengthen Your Recovery, a Pilates program following breast cancer surgery, a copy of the latest edition of The Beacon from B.C.N.A, information on how to order a My Journey Kit (I've already told you how good this resource is), and the Medicare External Breast Prostheses Reimbursement Program flyer.

This last inclusion, I will discuss further in the Reconstruction chapter.

Also included most importantly is a specially designed Berlei bra. This bra is shaped similar to a sports bra except it has pockets inside the cup, where a soft foam form is inserted to re-create the shape of a breast. I was so happy with this inclusion and I started wearing it about six weeks after the operation. It was awesome to look at myself in a top and see a shape that while not exactly the same as my last breast, was a pretty good imitation. The bra is lightweight and very comfortable. I wore mine for many years. Thankyou Berlei!!

As we made our way out of the office, I was apprehended by the Physiotherapist. She asked me to come into her office so she could check how things were progressing. I took off my shirt and the physio carefully looked at the scar and the tissue surrounding it. I told her about the pain I was getting underneath and along the inside of my arm, and after feeling around and up and down the arm, she announced that I had developed some Cording.

Cording, also known as Axillary web syndrome, can happen weeks or months after breast surgery, mastectomy or axillary surgery. It feels like a tight cord running from your armpit down the inner arm and is caused by hardened lymph vessels. Some people can see and feel raised cordlike structures across their arm, and these may restrict movement.

At least now I knew what was causing the pain and difficulty with moving my arm above my head and also out to the side. I would battle with this cording for many, many months. The physio also told me that I could start to gently massage the scar area and under my armpit. I was extremely hesitant to do this, as everything was still fresh in my mind. A journal entry from the 5th July: *"My baby and I miss snuggling in bed. My right side near the drain site is still tender and can't lay on that side. Chest wall is also tender and feels bruised to touch."*

However, the physio told me the importance of making sure I did the required exercises to keep the scar tissue from forming into a hard mass. I didn't want any long-term problems if I could be helping myself now. My armpit area was totally numb and I had an ultra-sensitivity along the entire back of my arm which was quite painful and annoying at times. It was then explained to me that the surgery site is much bigger than just where the breast had been removed from, as I had thought. As the breast tissue wraps around under the side of the chest and under the arm, the surgery site affects a large area of tissue and nerves. This was why I had discomfort in such a large area. Also, as I had the axillary clearance, the nerves from my armpit and reaching along my arm had also been somewhat affected. I hadn't expected this outcome. I think there was so much information to take in at diagnosis and so much to remember, that my brain may not have heard someone tell me about these things. I probably also read about them but couldn't remember. The massage was rather uncomfortable and the physio found the three cords within my arm. I was thankful for the massage later, as all the tissue had loosened and I felt better. Journal entry from 25th July: Have circled 4 ½ on the How am I feeling scale. *"Getting there. Have more energy. Still tender at back of arm and chest wall sometimes. Still can't lay on right side. Trying to massage chest and armpit as much as possible."* After spending about thirty minutes with the physio, Martin and I made our way to the Cancer Centre.

We arrived at the Cancer Centre and made our way to the desk clerk to check in. We were asked to take a seat in the Radiation waiting area. It was very confronting walking through the chemo waiting room. I felt quite nauseous and teary thinking, that might soon be me. I'm sure Martin felt the same way.

Shortly we were called up by a nurse who took us to the office of Dr. Joshua Dass. Martin and I entered and took a seat. There were introductions all around. Dr. Dass read through my history and we briefly discussed the operation and its outcomes.

My journal entry for this visit says it all: *"Saw the radiologist after being made an appointment. He said there was no reason to have radiotherapy as Dr. Kamyab had done a great job and removed lymph nodes and breast. Had a funny chat, laughed a lot with him and Martin. Got up and left REALLY HAPPY!! and relieved. Good day."* I felt so happy after this visit and I could tell Martin did too. We made our way home again. I was feeling happy, yet apprehensive about the upcoming treatment.

We received our appointment letter to see

the Oncologist via mail, about a week later. The appointment date was the 19th of July 2013. I was more anxious about this appointment as I knew some of the side effects of chemotherapy. While waiting for the day to come around, I again decided to be pro-active and arm myself with some knowledge of how other people had handled this often times debilitating treatment. I can't remember which website I visited back then, where I was reading stories from women who had experienced chemotherapy as an adjunct treatment to their surgeries. Even though I was reading such personal stories I didn't feel a sense of sadness or loss, I actually felt empowered. One story, in particular, led to me standing up and saying "That's what I'm going to do!" Read on.

The appointed day finally arrived and again Martin and I headed to the hospital in the car. We had our appointment at ten am in the Cancer Centre or the DD block. This always made me smile! We headed up in the lift to the waiting area and booked in with the clerk. I was taken into a small room by a nurse and weighed. This would happen before every appointment so that my weight could be monitored.

After this, I took a seat with Martin and we

waited to be called in. Looking around at the other people affected by Chemo, was a real in-your-face. There was no getting away from some of the side effects. I could see men and women from all walks of life and nationalities. Some had no hair, but still looked healthy. Others had no hair and didn't look quite as good. Some were displaying their lovely shiny bald domes, others wore colourful bandannas or beanies. There is no rule of thumb for cancer. It affects anyone. It was becoming more real to me as the minutes ticked by. There was a volunteer person from the Cancer Council of W.A. walking around and talking to those who didn't have anyone with them. I was so grateful I had my husband by my side.

After a short wait, my name was called by a nice looking young man. He introduced himself as Dr. Kelvin Siew. He was a Medical Oncologist. He led the way down a long corridor and into a small office. He sat down behind the desk and we took the seats opposite. Martin then introduced himself. Dr. Siew said that the meeting that day was to discuss what had happened to me so far, and what treatment regime I would be looking at. Another man then entered the room who introduced himself as Dr. Andrew Dean. He was a Consultant Oncologist. He said we would be in very good hands with Dr. Siew, and to ask any questions we had, to ensure we would get the most from the treatment. He then left the room and we continued with Dr. Siew.

The doctor started off by asking me about my general feeling of well-being and how I was feeling since the operation. Then we got down to business. He told me firstly, that I would probably lose my hair during the treatment. Martin and I looked at each other, as we already knew how we were going to deal with that.

As I mentioned earlier, during the wait for this appointment I had been doing some reading. These personal accounts told of how some women dealt with this treatment, its effects and how they had taken control. One such story touched me in a profound way. To make it personal, let's call this lady Jan (not her real name). Jan had started round one of her chemo regimes. For the next few weeks, Jan said she would wake up in the middle of the night and tug on her hair to see if it was falling out yet. After doing this for many nights consecutively, she had finally had enough. Jan said it was about three am when she woke one morning and thought to herself

"This is ridiculous. I'm not going to live like this." She then went into the bathroom, got some hair clippers from her bathroom cabinet and proceeded to shave her head! Jan took control. She said it was one of the only aspects of her treatment that she could control. After reading this, I went straight to Martin and said to him, "Listen to this. I want to do this too."

After looking at each other in the office, we relayed this story back to Dr. Siew and he said he had heard of people doing this, as a way to take control of their treatment. The doctor then told me I would be needing four rounds of chemo, starting on the 2nd of August. Each round would be given on a Friday, every three weeks. Before each round, I would need to have a blood test and on the appointment day, I would first see Dr. Siew to discuss the findings of the blood test and to see how I was feeling. Secondly, we would make our way downstairs to the treatment centre and have the chemotherapy administered. This could take anywhere from one and a half to two hours. He said depending on how I was feeling, I could continue to work, that was up to me. He also let me know that some people lose weight when having chemo, while others can put weight on. I was hoping a bit for the latter, it wouldn't hurt for me to lose a few kilos! Since my diagnosis, I had thought to myself, "If I want to have a muffin or a piece of cake, I'm going to because I don't know what the future holds!"

Dr. Siew then explained about the different drugs I would have. The first one was called Dexamethasone. This would be taken in combination with a drug called Docetaxel. These drugs are designed to slow the growth of, and hopefully destroy cancer cells. I was also told I would be taking a Hormone therapy called Tamoxifen, in the form of a tablet for the next five years. My breast cancer was later found to be Oestrogen and Progesterone receptor positive.

Hormone receptor-positive cancers need Oestrogen and/or Progesterone to grow and multiply. Hormone therapies such as Tamoxifen, target these hormones to stop them attaching to the cancer cells.

Dr. Siew also said he would give me a prescription for a small tablet called Zofran, which I could take if I felt nauseous etc. As it was very expensive, he had to call a government office to have the script approved. Martin and I tried to stay positive. We didn't know what the outcome would be, so we tried not to worry about things as they might not eventuate. Dr. Siew often looked at Martin and me in a funny way. I think this was because we could still have a laugh and tried not to upset ourselves unnecessarily. My journal entry from this day: *"Start chemo on 2/8. Trying not to think too much, but not knowing how I'll feel is the worst part. I don't want Martin and the kids to see me looking really sick. Pray for the best!"*

We were also told, that before the first round of chemo started, we would have to attend a group information session about chemotherapy. This would be held at the hospital and would take about one to one and a half hours and was compulsory. We couldn't start our treatment until we had completed the session.

Martin and I attended the session the following week. We arrived with many other people and arranged ourselves in the meeting room on the chairs provided. I can't remember who ran the session or much of what was spoken about. I do remember watching the DVD though. During the DVD many people spoke about their experience with chemo treatment and how it had affected their lives. They also shared some strategies for coping with the effects. At one point during the DVD, it finally hit me, like a bolt of lightning. F*##. I have to go through this. I am going to feel what these people feel and there's no way out. My family is going to have to watch me suffer the side effects of these nasty drugs. I remember tears came to my eyes and I felt a bit sick, but I didn't want to worry Martin, who was watching without showing much of how he felt. He is a Cancerian though, so he can sometimes bottle things up and keep his feelings hidden. At the end of the session, which was quite helpful, I guess, we had a cup of tea and then left for home.

As we now had a start date for the continuing treatment, I contacted my manager at work and again filled him in on the next step of the journey. I told him the start date of the Chemo treatment and what would happen over the next three months. I let him know that I expected to be able to continue working throughout this time.

"Let's just see how you go shall we?' These were his words, and never a truer word was said. He asked me to keep in touch with him after the treatment and let him know how I was going and we'd go from there.

I asked him if I could have Friday 2nd August

off for my first treatment. I fully expected to return to work on Monday morning, so I didn't plan anything else. As my bosses had not had any experience with a chemotherapy patient either, they went along with what I had asked for. I am still so grateful to my manager and the owners of the company that I worked for at the time, for the absolute compassion which was shown to Martin and I and our family during this trying time.

At the time of my diagnosis, we had been renting a house in the Perth hills suburb of Sawyers Valley. We had a large five-acre property which was filled with fruit trees. I had become quite the country kitchen cook, making jams and cookies using the fruit from the trees. However, the property was also a one hour drive, sometimes more depending on the traffic, from S.C.G.H. Martin and I had been seriously talking about a possible move since the mastectomy. We had been talking with our property manager about possibly getting out of the lease a few weeks early, so we could be moved into another property before my chemo treatment started. When we received the start date for the treatment, we got back in touch with the real estate manager and asked her to contact the owner and explain our situation. The manager called us back a couple of days later. She told us that the owner of the property was more than happy to let us leave the lease early and that he understood what we were going through. His own wife had been diagnosed with breast cancer and was currently undergoing treatment as well! Can you believe it? Our guardian angels were working overtime.

So we got the green light for the move. While I was recuperating from the mastectomy during the second week at home, I was busily looking for a new house to move to. I finally found one and asked my mum if she would come over and get me and we could drive down the hill to view it that afternoon. My doctor had suggested that I not drive for at least two to three weeks. Mum and I headed down the hill to Stratton and viewed a house there. I had my trusty and comfortable Zonta cushion with me. We put in an application for the house that day and heard from the property manager the following day, that the house was ours. Thank you, angels! Now, all we had to do was move.

We passed on the news to the family that we were on the move again. They understood our predicament and asked us if there was anything they could do. Well, my lovely brother and his even lovelier wife did more than most. They organised and paid for removalists to shift all our belongings to the new property. All we had to do was pack. We have moved a few times over the years, having been at the mercy of the rental market, so we were extremely proficient at it. On the 13th of July, we were in our new house which was now only thirty to thirty-five minutes from the hospital. I also jokingly added that we were now only 10 minutes from the Swan Districts hospital, in case we ever needed them. Remember those words folks!

My first chemotherapy treatment day arrived. Martin was not coming with me for this appointment, as he had already used up his carers leave and had used most of his annual leave days for the previous appointments he had attended with me. But I had my gorgeous mummy bear by my side. Before we went downstairs, I had to check in with the nurses and let them know I had arrived. Then I went around to a small room and was weighed and had my weight recorded in my notes. Then mum and I waited to be called by the doctor. I recall we only had to wait for about fifteen minutes, before being called by Dr.

Siew, who we followed down a corridor to his consulting room. He asked me how I was, told me my blood test results came back okay and that if I was ready to go, we could make our way downstairs to the treatment clinic. I said I was ready, so we said goodbye and made our way downstairs to the clinic.

Each visit to the clinic began with me scanning a little card the nurses gave me, which basically checks you in electronically. It saves a body having to sit there all day. Once I was checked in before each visit, I sat and waited for my name to be called. While I was waiting for my name to be called I looked around at all the other people that were there to have their chemo. There was a lot of us. I was a little bit apprehensive. I knew it wouldn't really hurt, as I had been a regular blood donor before I was diagnosed with Rheumatoid Arthritis. But as always, it's the fear of the unknown that keeps our stomachs turning and the butterflies flying. Mum was just sitting next to me taking it all in. We didn't really talk much. I think we both just wanted it to start and to know what was going to happen.

Finally, my name was called, so we followed the nurse into a large room that contained many reclining chairs, similar to a dentist chair but with bigger arms on the side. (I spoke to my mum last night on the phone after writing about this first chemo experience and she said she could remember exactly where we had sat). The nurse asked me all the standard questions to make sure I was the correct patient. She got the drip equipment ready with the trolley by her side. She asked me if I was comfortable and warm enough and I told her I was fine. Then we heard a loud voice say "Chemo!" During the entire time I had my treatment, I heard and became familiar with this voice. This nurse/orderly collected the patient's chemo drugs from the pharmacist and delivered them to the chemo clinic. So every time he entered with a new batch, he would repeat those words to let the nurses know he was there again.

After maybe a fifteen minute wait, my nurse brought over some bags of fluid and set about hooking them all up to the drip machine. Finally, as the nurse was inserting the needle into my vein, I looked across at my mum. She was crying. I know my mum would have gladly taken my place if she could have. I could see it in her eyes. As mothers, we never want our children to suffer.

It makes it harder when there is not a thing you can do to take away what is causing the suffering. The next few lines are for my mum;

"Mum, I want you to know that when I had you by my side, I felt loved and protected. I can't express my love and gratitude to you, for all you did for Martin and I and the kids, throughout the whole experience. When the needle finally entered my veins, to administer the drugs that would hopefully save my life, I saw your tears. It was finally real to you too. I didn't want you to see me suffer but you gladly sat with me and held my hand. Thank you, mum. I love you."

Once the drip had started, I sat back in the reclining chair. Mum covered me with the fluffy blanket that my aunt had given me, so I could snuggle under it. Mum sat by my side in the little cubicle space with a book. During the two hours it took to administer the chemo, we both were in our own worlds. I was flipping through a few magazines, mum was pretending to read her book! At some stage through the treatment, the nurses came around and offered me tea or coffee and some sandwiches, which I gladly took. Mum had brought her own snacks, so we had a little morning tea. Never did I think my mum and I would be having morning tea, while I had lifesaving chemotherapy drugs administered, but that's life sometimes. I had shared a lifetime of happiness and some sadness with my mum. Births, deaths, and marriages. And now here we were again, sharing a most unusual experience, but unfortunately now, not an uncommon one. I know there are many mothers, daughters, husbands and sons out there, going through exactly what we did. I hope they all have the wonderful support that I received, as I know this support helped me to have faith and hope that I would survive.

When the treatment was completed, all the equipment was taken away. The nurse asked me how I was and I replied that I felt okay. She then gave me a small card and told me to keep it with me. If I needed to see a doctor or go to the hospital, I should show them this card which had some details of my treatment written on it. Mum and I thanked the nurse and made our way out to the car. Mum asked me how I was feeling and I said I felt okay. So one down, three to go. While mum was driving carefully home, I called Martin to let him know everything had gone smoothly and that I felt okay. He was happy to hear from me and said he'd see me later at home.

Martin and I enjoy watching cooking shows. We also enjoy cooking dishes that are made on cooking shows. Masterchef was on T.V. at the time and I had printed a copy of Maggie Beers (don't you just love her) Slow-braised Beef cheeks in Barossa Shiraz. I had been wanting to make this dish for ages, and so I thought that since I had the Friday off from work, that once my treatment had finished, I could go home and make the dish for dinner that night. Idiot!!! Mum and I arrived home and I set about preparing the ingredients for the dish. I spent a lovely afternoon lovingly caring for my beautiful beef cheeks and looking forward to dinnertime. Mum was just as excited as I was, as, like us, she thoroughly enjoys her food. A couple of times during the afternoon, mum commented on the red blotches on my neck. I told her they were there as I was hot from cooking. Martin arrived home later in the afternoon and soon we were dishing up for dinner. This was about six thirty pm.

We laid the plates on the table and Martin and mum proceeded to tuck into the dish with a lot of mmmm's and ah's. I started to eat but my appetite seemed to have diminished over the afternoon. I poked the food around my plate for a while but I was pleased that Martin and mum were enjoying their dinner. However, my neck had started to get a bit itchy and I felt tired and didn't really feel all that well.

Towards the end of the meal, mum said: "Carry, look at your face and neck, it's all red and blotchy."

Martin agreed with her, so I got up and went to our ensuite bathroom for a closer look. Oh, it sure was red and blotchy. By that stage, I had started to get itchy on my hands, as well as my neck and face. I sat on the side of my bed and took out the leaflet that I had been given about the chemo drugs I had received. I was specifically reading about the side effects of the drugs and what to look out for. As I read down the list, I shouted out to Martin and Mum.

"I think I'm having an allergic reaction and it says that we should probably go to the hospital."

Now, remember a few paragraphs back, I mentioned we had just moved into a new house and that it was only about a ten minute drive from the Swan Districts Hospital? I really felt as though I was being divinely cared for. Whether it was God or my guardian angels, I was extremely grateful for the support.

We asked mum to stay and look after the children, while Martin and I headed for the hospital. By this stage, my throat had become itchy and I was feeling as though it was becoming constricted. I was trying to stay calm, while asking Martin to step on it!

We arrived at the hospital with Martin dropping me at the Emergency entrance and then going to find a parking spot. I entered the doors and went straight up to the Triage nurse who took one look at me, as I handed her the card the nurses at S.C.G.H had given me and quickly took my Medicare card. She took a few details and then rushed me into the emergency room. As there was a shortage of beds, I was put in a wheelchair and by this time my feet had started going numb. I was seen by a doctor after maybe five to ten minutes, who asked me a load of questions and then suggested I was having an allergic reaction to one of the chemotherapy drugs. Thank you, Doctor, I concur. I was finally offered a bed and a nurse came and inserted a needle into my arm to administer some Phenergan. I was also given a tablet of Ranitidine. After about ten to fifteen minutes, the symptoms finally started easing one by one. I was told I could go home about forty-five minutes later, with instructions to cease taking the Dexamethasone tablets and to take a Zofran tablet if I was feeling nauseous instead.

The following morning I had another 2 Phenergan tablets, as my face and chest were still very hot and flushed. A journal entry for the 3/8: *"Slept all day. Very thirsty. Feel quite yukky. My forearm aches where the needle for the chemo went in. I'm going to call Oncology Monday morning and see what they say."* So I had quite an eventful start to my chemo regime.

On the Sunday morning after a good sleep, I mentioned to Martin again, the fact that I wanted to shave my head and not be forced to watch my hair fall out. As we wanted to include the children, I went and asked them if they would like to watch Martin shave my head. Tyson replied that he didn't want to, however, Jade said she would like to come and watch. We went outside and sat at the outdoor setting. Martin had a set of clippers and a pair scissors.

"Are you ready?" he asked me.

I looked across at Jade. She was just calmly looking at me and smiling. I didn't know how she was feeling, as she tends to play her emotional cards close to her chest. I haven't brought up what happened to me very often, as I feel that going through it once, was probably enough for my children.

"I'm ready," was my reply.

I did not lament the loss of my hair for one second. For me, this move became my symbol of control and I was extremely happy to have this one small victory. I did not want my family to see my hair falling out bit by bit. I told my friends and family that I never wanted to look like a mis-used dolly. So, as Martin began to cut my hair shorter and then finally to shave the rest from my scalp, as each strand fell away, I felt stronger mentally. Journal entry for 4/8: *"Jade came out to watch Martin cut my hair and then shave my head. It went really well. Have a killer sore throat on the right side and a painful left hip joint. Just feel a bit weak."*

I will include a few journal entries for the week following my first chemo treatment, as a lot happened.

Journal entry Monday 5/8: *"Went to see Doc. Throat was so sore. Maybe the beginning of an ulcer in my throat. On antibiotics for the week. Not working Monday or Tuesday. Sleeping every day for two to three hours. Very tired.*

Thursday 8/8: *"No work this week, too tired. Broke a corner of my tooth tonight, picking a cracker out of my tooth but instead of cracker got a tooth! Had tooth fixed on 9/8. On antibiotics for another week. Had a tight chest."*

Saturday 10/8: *"Have a very funny chest and coughing. Took my puffer today but still feels like I'm getting a cold. Jade has been sick since 8/8 on antibiotics and steroids. Tried to keep away from her and asked her to stay in her room the whole time. Hope it doesn't come to anything."*

Monday 12/8: *"Bugger- Got a nasty cold now. Full of coughing, blocked nose. Went to the doc. Having a week off work again to rest and keep warm. Oh Dear!*

Friday 16/8: *"Feeling better. Cold easing off. Hopefully back to work Monday!! Looking forward to it a lot. Just have to remember to rest. Sat/Sun- Had a bloody fantastic weekend, with movies and casino!!*

Two weeks after my first chemo treatment: Monday 19/8: *"Felt great. Went back to work till Thurs 22/8. Got a bit tired as the week went on but felt totally normal. Work, cook tea WOW!!*

So no sooner had I managed to get through the first chemo treatment, than the second one came on the 23rd of August. My good friend Robyn had offered to take me for my second appointment. So I thanked my mum for her offer to take me, as I thought it was important to allow other family and friends to be involved, if they wanted to.

In April of that year, Martin and I had helped with some catering for the 21st birthday party of one of Robyn's children. We didn't get our diagnosis until May. As I had only told the immediate family about my diagnosis initially, Robyn hadn't known about it. However, word gets around. A young lady who was close to our family and had already been told our news, also worked with Robyn's daughter and so one day, my name was brought up in the conversation, which was then passed on to Robyn. She then slyly arranged to meet up with me, on the pretence of returning a plastic container that we had left behind at the party. A few days later, we sat down together, after ordering our coffee.

"So how are you, Caroline?" Robyn asked.

"I'm okay thanks Robyn, how are you?" was my reply.

"No, how ARE you, Caroline?" Robyn asked again, in a somewhat firmer voice.

With this second line of questioning, and the look on my friends face, I knew Robyn had somehow received our news.

"Alright, who told you?' I asked.

Robyn then related the story to me. We sat together, while I told her about the diagnosis so far and what would be happening in a few weeks. She told me then, if there was anything her or her husband could do for us, to just let them know. Robyn and I had known each other for almost fifteen years at that stage. I had worked for her and her husband for many years previously and we had stayed in touch. I was quite surprised when Robyn offered to take me to any appointments that I needed help with, as we didn't live in each other's pockets. Sometimes the help you need comes from unexpected places. I was really happy to have a friend coming along with me. I know it was very confrontational for Robyn to witness my treatment. Thank you, Robyn, your compassion meant so much to Martin and I.

My family always supported me on Chemo day. Every third Friday, I'd receive text messages from my brother and his wife, my sister and my niece, with good wishes and lovely messages of support and love. Than you family, for your wonderful heartfelt messages and support!

As I never drove myself to the chemo treatment days, Robyn offered to pick me up and take us in. I gave her a time to pick me up and she was usually always on time. When she finally arrived, she told me that a car had run up the rear end of her car, as she was waiting to join traffic. I felt so bad. If she hadn't been coming to help me, her car wouldn't be damaged. She said not to worry about it, but I thought to myself, why did that have to happen when she was doing a good turn for someone?

We arrived at the hospital without incident and followed the same routine as the last visit. I was checked in upstairs, weighed and then saw the doctor. Due to the allergic reaction I had suffered from the last chemo drug Docetaxel, the doctor said I would be receiving a new one, called Doxorubicin. He was hoping that I would be able to have this one with no reaction. He asked me how I was feeling, so I gave him the run down from the previous round. After a short visit, we left his office.

Robyn and I then headed downstairs to the

clinic and checked in. We were called in shortly by the nurses. I was seated again in a reclining chair and the nurse set up all the equipment required. The nurse had to use a different place on my arm for the cannula, as they were not allowed to go higher than the last place the needle had been. A vein was finally found near my wrist and the infusion began. At one point during the treatment, my hand that had the needle in it began hurting really badly. The nurse got me a heat pack to place over my hand which seemed to help. However, the pain still continued so I called the nurse over and when we took the heat pack off my hand, we could see the drug inside all the little veins on the top of my hand. It looked like a pink roadmap. She quickly went and told a colleague of hers and together they came back and checked my hand. They then made the decision to stop the treatment for a short while. I think Robyn was quietly freaking out a bit, I know I was.

This incident was known as Tracking and it was quite common. The nurse came back and gave me some Phenergan which helped. I could slowly see the pink roadmap disappear. After about half an hour, the drip was started again and we continued without any problems. I had also been told that with the chemo drug they had given me this time, when I went to the toilet I might notice that my urine may be bright pink. I knew what they meant a short while after, as I needed to relieve myself and Lo and Behold there was my bright pink urine. This chemo round took about three and a half hours. Robyn patiently waited in the little cubicle by the side of my chair. What a lovely friend! After the round was finished, we finally made our way out to the car and Robyn drove me home. I thanked her and told her once again how sorry I was about her car. Thank you, Robyn, for supporting me through a difficult day xx.

My journal entry for the 23/8: *"Started Doxorubicin & Cyclo with Dex. After felt quite tired for the rest of the day and quite fuzzy in the head. Went to bed at 7 pm- didn't feel like tea. Had a yoghurt. Had cotton mouth tonight."*

One of the side effects of some chemo drugs is Cottonmouth. It was such a weird feeling. Basically, there was no saliva or moisture left in my mouth and I felt as if I had a large ball of cotton wool in my mouth. Even drinking water didn't help much. I remembered hearing or reading about it previously, but until it happened, I had forgotten about it. There are many side effects that can occur, but as each of us is different, it becomes a bit like Lotto. Some win, others don't.

With each chemo treatment that I had, for the week following, I was wiped out. I couldn't go to work, as I developed "Chemo fog or brain", which is another wonderful side effect. My mind just turned to mush pretty much and as I was working in foreign money exchange, I thought it best if I didn't go to work. Thank goodness for Martin and my Journal calendar. As the days progressed from the treatment day on a Friday, I became progressively more tired and unable to think. I spent my days in a haze of sleep and nausea. That's all I could manage to do well. Sleep. The Zofran I had been given for nausea, worked amazingly well though and usually within a short while after taking it, the nausea would have subsided. When I reached Wednesday's, I always seemed to get weepy. Martin would come home from work, and there I'd be lying in bed and I'd start crying and telling him I was sorry he had to do everything and he'd give me a cuddle and say it wasn't my fault. We just had to do what we had to do. By the following Friday, my son would begin to recognise me again and say "Yeh, mum's back."

Martin said recently, it's as though someone flicked a switch and from one day to the next, I was back. I only notice now that I am writing this book and referring to my journal, that I didn't write much at all during the time of my chemo treatment. I think it probably has something to do with the chemo fog and basically being unable to think for the week. When I finally came 'back', I just wanted to join in with life again and do all the things I usually did, but couldn't during that foggy week of treatment.

My wonderful husband looked after me, the children, the house, the bills, the shopping and went to his full-time job every day, without complaint. Mum helped Martin where she could and my family pitched in with a meal or two. But on the whole, it was the love of my life, that took me from one end of the deep dark tunnel to the other end. And he still managed to make me laugh!

I was really glad that we had cut my hair off though, as even though we had done that, the inside of my little white cotton hat that I used to sleep in, was covered in little hairs which gradually became less, the more treatments I had. I had shopped online for a really nice hat to wear once my hair was gone. I couldn't seem to find one I liked in the few shops I looked in, but I found a really great site called Hat show. They are in S.A. So I purchased a nice cotton stretch Chemo hat, with scarf attached and also the plain cotton hat to wear to bed.

For many years, I had bought a Canteen bandanna on Bandanna Day, which raises money to provide services for young people who have, or have a family member who has cancer. I had quite a nice collection and now wore them during my own cancer journey.

I did receive a voucher from the hospital to purchase a wig. I went to a shop called Curly Sue and the lovely lady there helped me to find a wig, similar to the style my hair had been before the chemo. When I tried it on and turned to Martin, he had tears in his eyes and told me I looked exactly how I used to! Needless to say, we bought that one. I still have it at home and it's in new condition, as I always found it too hot to wear. I preferred a bandanna or the stretch hat, as it was cooler for me.

Before my chemo treatment started I had read that it was helpful to have a range and variety of foods available as you never knew what you might feel like eating, if anything. So Martin and I had shopped and bought a wide variety of food that we felt I might like during my treatment weeks. Two of the best things I ate over the three months of treatment were Cauliflower fritters and Chicken Noodle Soup.

My wonderful friend Rachelle, who I first met when our boys were together in kindy, had bought a book for me titled "What to eat during Cancer treatment" by Jeanne Besser. This book was so great. It was divided up into sections that related to the side effects of treatment and what you could eat to alleviate them. For example, there was a section on foods to eat if you had Nausea, Constipation or a Sore mouth etc. Well, I can tell you that Martin made those Cauliflower fritters in bulk and cooked that soup every week! They were both very simple to make. I used to put a little tomato relish on top of the fritters and heat them for about 15 seconds in the microwave. They were my go to, when I didn't know what I felt like eating. The soup was so light in texture but had a lovely depth of flavour. It's funny but when I think about them now, I wouldn't want to have them. If you want to offer something for a friend or family member, this book was invaluable.

Once my treatment was finished, I took the book along with me and left it at the Solaris Cancer centre at S.C.G.H. They have books that people can take and read or use when they are having their cancer treatment. I wanted someone else to have the benefit of the book just as I had. Thanks a million for the terrific book, Rachelle!

For the third chemo treatment on the 13th September, mum was present again. Martin had asked his boss if he could attend the fourth and final one with me and his boss had agreed. Mum and I went through the same process as in the previous two treatments. This third treatment went quite smoothly and I only had a minor reaction which disappeared quite quickly. Again for the week following treatment, my day's involved sleep, nausea, and tears. But again by Friday, I was back to my old self. I did gradually become a bit weaker as the treatment went on, but I still managed to become more like my old self each time.

I obviously wasn't looking my best during this time either, but I was still going to work for two out of the three weeks. My wonderful work colleague Peng, was so supportive and encouraging. She saw me every day and never judged what I looked like, and some days were pretty scary!! She carried the workload and always made sure we had a laugh during the day. It was awesome to feel 'normal' during these times and I really appreciated everything Peng and my bosses did for me during a rather tough year. A big kiss and hug for you Peng. mwa xx.

My fourth and final chemo treatment, was on the 4th October 2013. Two days before my birthday. My hubby was finally with me and we made our way to the hospital. When we were called into the doctor's office, we had a good laugh with Dr. Siew and thanked him for being so nice and happy and positive. He gave me my prescription for the Tamoxifen, which I would take for the next five years and wished us good luck. We didn't need to see him anymore, after this day.

Once we were seated downstairs in the clinic, a nurse told me that I would be having some Phenergan first, which she would give me intravenously, before the chemo drugs were given. I thought that was a good idea and so did Martin. The treatment went well and finished in good time. We thanked the nurses in the clinic for all their care and made our way out to the car. What a relief it was to know we had come out the other end. I was so happy that the treatment had finished.

I had organised for my family to visit me to have a birthday/end of chemo party! We waited until the following Saturday and we had a lovely party. I had bought a bright pink wig from Kmart to wear. My family hadn't seen me since I had lost my hair and I didn't want it to be too confrontational for them. While everyone was arriving, I walked out in my pink wig but later on, I got a bit hot and itchy in it so I took it off, giving them their first look at my bald dome. We took photos for a laugh and I said I wanted everyone to have a photo taken with me, with the person wearing the pink wig! Boy did we have a laugh. All my lovely family members had a photo taken in the wig. It was a special day and a birthday party I'll never forget.

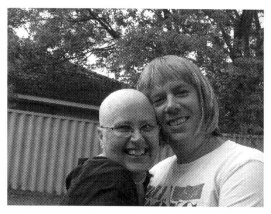

Martin and I getting in on the action
at my 45th birthday party.

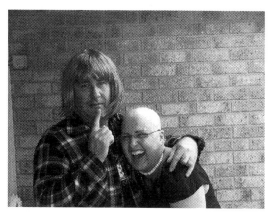

My brother John. Always makes the family laugh.
Just what the doctor ordered at this party!

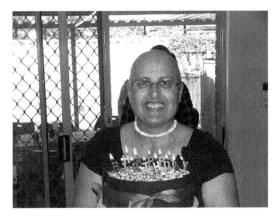

The Birthday girl. It was so good to see all my family together after a pretty rough few months. It felt great to be doing 'normal' again.

Martin's perspective on Treatment

Dealing with the news that someone you love has been diagnosed with this nasty disease is one thing. Living with someone going through the treatment is a whole new ball game. You enter a world that is completely foreign to you and even though you listen to the doctors and nurses and all of the other people giving you the information, you still have that little voice in the back of your head saying, What is all of this about? Here we were plodding along in our life, having a good time, watching our children grow up, planning for the future, then along comes something that threatens to take it all away. There is talk of operations, chemotherapy, side-effects, hospital visits, doctor's visits and a myriad of other things you have to take into account, when all you want to happen is for it all to go away and get back to what you thought was normal. Unfortunately, this became normal for some time.

I must admit that I do have some trouble remembering the details of the last 5 years. Caroline has asked me "Do you remember?" ......

117

quite a lot while writing this book but quite a few of the details have vanished from my memory. As mentioned before, I am prone to sticking my head in the sand but I think this comes more from self-preservation and making sure that I could still function to ensure that the family got through what-ever was to be thrown at us.

Caroline has said quite a lot about how I was during this stage and that I was her rock etc. But believe me, she was the one who got us through all of this. Her positive attitude, her worrying about everyone but herself, her strength and her down right stubbornness that she was going to get through this thing, gave me the strength to get through it.

I can totally understand Caroline's desire to shave her head to stop her hair falling out but it would have to be one of the worst things I have ever had to do in my life. Seeing her without hair, was a hundred times worse than seeing her missing one, or eventually both breasts. I can easily look at a picture of her "flat" chest but every time I see a picture of her with no hair, it upsets me big time.

Caroline was so worried that my feelings for her would change, when she was missing a breast or even after she had the reconstruction. I didn't marry her boobs. I married her as a package. Yes, her breasts did hold some benefits for me, but she is still the same loving person that I married.

Going through Chemo was hard. Poor me having to work and cook and clean and do the washing, while my wife lounged around in bed expecting mountains of cauliflower fritters and litres of chicken noodle soup!!!!! Seeing her react to the chemo the way she did, was very distressing when you take into account the way she normally is – a mountain of energy that will do everything she can to help others, reduced to a sleepy, crying, apologetic zombie. Then comes the day that the switch is flicked and back she came. It was quite amazing the difference from morning to night. I always looked forward to that day, as it was the day I got my wife back.

One thing I have learned from all of this, is sometimes you will only get help if you ask. I pretty much decided to take on everything myself and not ask anyone for anything. I am sure that if I had asked anyone for help, I would have received it but Mr. Stubborn is not one to ask. I took on a lot and never complained about having to do any of it but it did wear me down.

Something I have been told a number of times is, I was going through this as well. Not physically, but emotionally. If I had to go through all of this again, (and believe me I hope I never do) I would make sure that I got some help and talked a bit more and asked family and friends for help. Caroline's mum was always there when I needed her help and I am sure if I had asked, she would have done more.

My way of dealing with the operations was to have a routine. My employers did not want me at work the days Caroline was operated on, so I always managed to be with her. Leaving her when she was heading into the operating theatre was always hard and even though you know she is going to be in the best of care, the little "what if" voice gets me every time. I did the same thing during all operations. I headed to a restaurant, had food and usually a beer, read my book and tried to not think about what was happening. I would then head back to the hospital after a couple of hours and wait. As most of Caroline's operations were in the afternoon, I found a waiting room that was generally deserted by about 3 pm that I would set myself up in, with a book and a drink and a snack, to wait to see Caroline before I went home.

It was hard not going with Caroline to all of her Chemo treatments and missing the occasional doctor's appointments but my employer was being very fair and I didn't want to rock the boat too much, as I was still on probation and really liked the job and wanted to stay. I always insisted that Caroline ring me if I missed anything, to give me a full rundown on how it went.

Chapter 3

Reconstruction

I was ready for this stage. After having the first mastectomy and subsequent chemotherapy from June 2013 through until October 2013, I now allowed my body time to heal. I also allowed my mental and emotional state, time and space to breathe. We had all been through so much, from diagnosis through to the treatments and it had all taken its toll. Maybe not that anyone else could see. I believe we sometimes tend to see the outer happenings of those around us and forget about the inner. Our friends and family knew we had had the mastectomy and the chemotherapy treatment. For them, it may have seemed to be all over. For Martin and I, however, we faced what we had been through every day. Whenever my husband saw my poor scarred flat chest, and whenever I looked into the bathroom mirror, the reminder was there, of just what we had faced. It was easy for me, to have the breast removed. As I have mentioned previously, I just wanted cancer taken from my body. If that meant losing the breast so be it. Living with the consequences of that choice, however, was something else entirely. I will talk more about things of this nature in the next chapter Rebuilding. Needless to say, I was chafing at the bit to restore my chest to something that resembled what I had been born with.

I called S.C.G.H in early January 2014 and left a message for Dr. Kamyab at the Breast Clinic, to request an appointment to discuss a prophylactic mastectomy. Not everyone chooses to have a prophylactic mastectomy. It is a deeply personal choice. It was, however, one that I had made as soon as I knew I had to have the initial mastectomy. I knew right away, that I would want the other breast off as well. I did not want to give cancer any chance to appear in my remaining breast. The clinic nurses told me they would pass on the message and that I would receive an appointment letter as usual in the mail. I received the letter a few weeks later with an appointment date of 13th January 2014.

During the months following the initial mastectomy, I wore the Berlei bra that had been given to me by the nurses at the S.C.G.H breast clinic. It was wonderful to have the soft form shape in the place of my right breast, however, as there was no weight to the form, I still felt as though I was missing something. Included in the kit from Berlei, is a flyer explaining the Medicare External Breast Prostheses program. A few months after the mastectomy, I decided to read the flyer to find out about the program and what it entailed. I didn't really understand what breast prosthesis was, or what it would look like. After reading the flyer I was extremely excited. The program assists people in the cost of external breast prostheses. There are certain criteria that you need to meet such as being enrolled in Medicare and needing breast surgery as a result of breast cancer. I had ticked all the boxes for eligibility, so I called the wonderful team at Breast Cancer Care W.A. who told me about a company called Breast Care W.A.

This company specialises in after-surgery garments for men and women. I went straight to their website and searched for external prostheses and they had some available. I made an appointment with them the following day and went along to the store to have my fitting.

When I arrived the lovely ladies asked me questions about the style of bra I wanted and I was then taken into a fitting room. I told the lady that I wanted a prosthesis and she showed me one. It was amazing! The form is made of silicone so even though it has the weight it also has softness. I was shown a variety of lovely post-surgery bras and finally chose a nice black one. The bras are similar to the Berlei soft form bra, in that they have internal pockets to insert the prostheses. The lady showed me how to insert the silicone form. I then took off my soft form bra and was helped into the new bra. It was unbelievable!!! It felt like I still had my right breast. The weight of the prostheses almost mimicked my old breast. I was so happy. This bra not only looked pretty, but it also made me feel 'normal' again. I was looking at myself in the mirror, turning this way and that admiring my new chest. The ladies were very happy for me and I just felt wonderful. I'm pretty sure the reimbursement from Medicare just about covered the entire cost of the form. There are many available, so depending on the one you choose, there may be some out of pocket expense.

Well worth it though. Now armed with my new found confidence, I set off to see Dr. Kamyab on the 13th of January to discuss the next operation.

On arriving at the clinic I again went through the arrival process and made my way into the clinic waiting area. I waited a short time and was then ushered into Dr. Kamyab's office, again with a breast care nurse present. We had a great chat about how the chemo had gone and how I had been feeling for the past few months. I told Dr. Kamyab that I was excited and very keen for the next mastectomy. Dr. Kamyab said that she was going to refer me to one of her colleagues, Dr. Kallyani Ponniah, for the next mastectomy and subsequent reconstruction. The breast clinic staff would organise the appointment for me as usual. Even though I was sounding very positive, Dr. Kamyab said it was a normal procedure for people electing to have a prophylactic mastectomy, to have a chat with a clinical psychologist. I would need to have this appointment before the surgery. I told the doctor that I was more than happy to see the psychologist and she said she would organise the appointment for me. The purpose of my consultation with the psychologist was to discuss the psychological implications associated with the treatment plan for the left side mastectomy and the bilateral breast implant reconstruction.

My visit with Dr. Kamyab was soon over and I thanked her very much for helping me and caring so much about my welfare. I was looking forward to meeting my new surgeon.

During the time I waited for my appointments to be sent in the mail, I looked through the booklets that I had received in the My Journey Kit. There is a wealth of helpful information in the two booklets, and as I wanted to find out more about the types of reconstruction available, I read them every minute I could.

Now again, the choice to have any reconstruction at all is a personal choice. Some women choose implants, either Silicone or Saline. This was going to be my choice. Others choose to have the breast reconstructed from their own breast tissue. The tissue is taken from places like your tummy, thigh or back in the form of a flap (see chapter 4). I have a friend in Japan who chose to have her breast reconstructed using a flap technique, as she said she wanted to use her own cells. While others make the choice not to have any reconstruction done at all, or the surgery is delayed, sometimes for many years. Until I had spoken to Dr. Ponniah though, I was going to keep an open mind. I trusted the opinions of the doctors trying to help me.

I finally received the appointment letter to see Dr. Ponniah, and Martin and I went to the breast clinic again on the 12th February 2014. I was really excited about the operation and to meet the doctor. I also wanted to find out which implants I would be having. Martin said he didn't have any opinion as to what he thought I should have. As always, he said he was just happy to have me. The type of implants I chose wasn't going to bother him at all, it was my choice. We got to the hospital and went up to the breast clinic. My name was called after a short wait and we were shown into the office.

Dr. Ponniah introduced herself and we did also. She then briefly went through my history and we discussed what I wanted to happen next. Dr. Ponniah showed us some implants and explained the difference between Silicone and Saline. I chose Silicone implants as they have a nice natural look and feel. I chose round high profile implants as I thought they would suit me and I had looked at pictures of implants and thought those looked nice. It's very hard to choose something like implants. Also, as I had lost a lot of breast tissue with the first mastectomy, I didn't know what the finished product would look like. Dr. Ponniah then explained the initial reconstruction process.

Firstly, I would have the left breast removed. During the same operation, I would have tissue expanders inserted under the pectoral muscle and skin of each side of my chest. At the same time, the expanders would then be filled with one hundred ml of a saline solution which would be filled through a small port at the top of the expander. That would be the first step. Following this step, I would be expected to visit the clinic every three to four weeks to have another one hundred ml inserted into each expander until there was approximately four hundred ml in each side. This process would slowly stretch the muscle and skin so that the breast implants could be inserted later. Once the expanders had four hundred ml in each side, I would have another operation to exchange the expanders for the silicone implants. Dr. Ponniah also suggested I have two weeks off work following the operation to recuperate and also possibly not to drive if I could. I wanted to do everything I could to help myself so I readily agreed. The doctor said it should be quite a straightforward operation. I would be in the hospital anywhere from four to six days depending on the volume of the drainage bottles, just like the first mastectomy. I really liked Dr. Ponniah straight away.

Both Martin and I felt really comfortable with her and she was able to put our minds at ease. My opinions were always listened to and my questions thoroughly answered. I felt safe and in good hands. The doctor checked her surgery schedule and asked me if Friday 11th April would suit us to have the operation. Well, I was so happy!! Only a couple of months to wait and the next phase of our journey would start. I was really excited. Dr. Ponniah filled out all the necessary paperwork for the operation and I signed on the dotted line, so to speak. I would receive the pre-admission and surgery details in the mail. We thanked Dr. Ponniah and left with big grins on our faces. I think Martin was as excited as I was, although I feel his excitement was more for me, than for himself.

During the wait for the next surgery, I had my appointment with the psychologist from S.C.G.H, on 28th February. It was a very informal meeting.

The psychologist and I discussed my feelings on the cancer diagnosis and how I had handled it. I was also asked general health and well- being questions associated with my recovery so far and also about future operations and recovery. I later received a copy of the report which was also sent to my first surgeon. It basically described the points we had discussed at our meeting and how I was feeling about the upcoming surgery. It was quite funny for me to note that at the end of the letter, the psychologist states that she feels I am quite comfortable doing external activity relevant to my need, but possibly less comfortable engaging in restful activity which might provide restorative opportunities for my body! Wow, how did she read me that well in such a short session? I did sometimes have trouble taking "me time", however, Martin ensured I took the time to relax and recuperate after each surgery. So now that the psychologist box was ticked, we could go ahead with the operation.

I was booked in for pre-admission on the 3rd April at the Day of Surgery clinic. This appointment was again to check blood work, meet with the anaesthetist and have height and weight measured again. Also, a quick chat with a colleague of Dr. Ponniah's just to make sure all the details were correct and that everything else was good to go. Obviously, they check if you have been feeling well and healthy, so these pre-operative checks are very important for your health and also the health of those around you. I mentioned to Martin that I would attend this appointment on my own, as we knew what would occur and there didn't seem the need for him to take time off work again to sit around the clinic and wait to be seen. I knew he liked to be with me for appointments but sometimes I had to put my foot down and say no! Everything went smoothly at the appointment and I left after a couple of hours, really excited for the upcoming operation in a week.

The following day Friday 4th April I was starting work later in the day, as I had a wedding to attend in the morning. I have mentioned in a previous chapter that I have Rheumatoid Arthritis. Sometimes you can have what is called a 'flare". This is where some of the symptoms of pain, swelling, and fatigue, can be greatly enhanced. I believe with the running around I was doing to appointments and also feeling a bit anxious about the surgery, that this caused my body to retaliate. I woke that morning feeling absolutely exhausted, but I really wanted to go to the wedding of one of our family friends.

So I pushed myself to get up and get dressed and start the day. I attended the lovely wedding and had just enough time to stop in for a small chat and something to eat at the reception, before I had to head into work. I arrived at work and started my shift. Halfway through my shift, I felt the straps on my sandals were really tight. I mentioned this to my colleague Peng, before turning my chair to the side and lifting up my work trouser leg. We both looked down at my legs, horrified. The area from my knees to my ankles was extremely swollen. Peng and I looked at each other and then Peng said she thought I better see a doctor. I agreed.

I left work and went to see a doctor at my local surgery. I told him what had been happening. He suggested that I should have a week off work before the operation to just relax and that I should elevate my legs as much as possible. I called my manager and Peng to let them know. I felt bad about not being able to work, however, I knew my health had to come first. Thank goodness the swelling went down over the week, so by the time the operation day came around, they were back to normal.

On the 11th April 2014, Martin and I again headed into the hospital for the next round of surgery. This time I had a small bag packed with everything I would need for my four to six-day stay. Remember if you have to stay in a hospital to bring things such as earplugs, headphones and of course your phone charger. Martin was always so good at reminding me of these things. I also followed my own advice about taking Metamucil for the week preceding the operation and it worked a treat. No constipation this time. A journal entry for the day: *My baby and I are taking turns crying and laughing. Feel quite nervous. We know what's coming, well some of it! Luv ya babe xx*

We were at the hospital at 6.30am and after collecting the paperwork from the clerks downstairs, we headed up to the Day of Surgery ward. We waited in the seats just outside the waiting room as they were quite big chairs and I was able to curl up with a blanket and stay warm and comfortable until I was called in.

During the wait to be called, a young medical student called Jess approached me. She told me what she was doing at the hospital and then asked me if she could ask me some questions about my treatment etc. She then asked if she could come and watch the operation and see me during my stay at the hospital. I was happy to help her and so I agreed that it would be fine. She was quite excited, as she had never seen my kind of operation before. She said goodbye and that she would see me later.

As we were sitting just outside the waiting room, we couldn't always hear what was going on inside the waiting room itself. As the public hospital system is very busy and emergency operations have to be done, sometimes patients have their operations cancelled to be re-scheduled. On the day of my operation, two people had to have emergency surgery. We overheard some people talking and they were very frustrated as they had had their surgery cancelled for that day, after having waited for two hours. I looked at Martin and said I hoped mine would not be cancelled. Thankfully after a short time, I was called into the waiting room and the process of getting ready for surgery started again.

My wonderful husband Martin, was again by my side while we waited for the surgery time to approach. We had a quick kiss every now and again and held hands and chatted about what he was going to do while I was in surgery. As before, my hubby didn't want to have anything to eat, as he didn't like to eat as I couldn't. I knew he was getting hungry, because I could hear his tummy rumbling. We were told the surgery could take two and a half hours, so Martin was going to go into Subiaco to have some lunch and maybe a beer!! He deserved at least a couple.

The orderly came to get me for surgery at 2.45pm. Martin gave me a big kiss and left, saying he would see me later that day. The orderly pushed me through the back corridors of the hospital, into what I call the "waiting bay" of the operating theatre. While we were waiting for the theatre to be ready, the anaesthetist came and inserted a cannula into my vein. The medical student Jess joined us and we chatted for a few minutes, until everything was ready to go.

Once we were in the operating theatre, I was helped on to the skinny little operating table and everybody did their thing. A blood pressure cuff was put on my left arm, warm blankets were placed over my body and the anaesthetist asked me if I was ready. Dr. Ponniah arrived and said hello and asked how I was feeling. I told her I was ready to go and quite excited. The anaesthetist then told me he was going to place a mask over my mouth and that he wanted me to take a few slow, deep breaths. He placed the mask over my mouth and as I was taking my slow deep breaths and he was telling me what a good job I was doing, I noticed the lights on the ceiling, looked very much like the dance floor from the movie scene in Saturday Night Fever!

I thought I was just thinking this to myself. But no. My crazy anaesthetic filled mind, had actually voiced these thoughts out loud, as I was drifting into unconsciousness. How do I know this you may ask? Well, a few days later when I was in the general ward, I had a visit from Jess, the medical student. She asked me how I was and how I felt the operation had gone. She then told me that she had heard something very funny, while I was being put under. She said I kept mumbling about 'disco lights' and 'dance floors'!! Hahaha. I then told her what I had been thinking about and we both had a great laugh. Ah, anaesthetics can be fun sometimes, can't they?

After the operation, I was taken to the recovery ward and later around 8 pm, I was then taken to the day surgery ward for the night. A journal entry: *"Couldn't use bedpan at ten pm so tried to go to the toilet. Couldn't walk so used commode chair. Vomited when I got there. Had to go toilet again later. Again used commode chair but vomited again. Had eaten a ½ curried egg sandwich. Felt ok, bit stiff. Gave me painkiller under the tongue. It was lovely to look down and see two matching sides. I made the right decision! My lovely nurse (tea & biscuits) was there again. Ahhhh….Liz, I think."*

The following day I was taken up to the general medical ward, seventy-one, around twelve pm. My room, seventeen B, contained four beds. I had two drains on the left side and one in my right side. There was now one hundred millilitres in each expander.

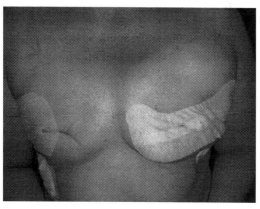

The picture above was taken seven days post-op. The curved scar on the right-hand side, is from the first mastectomy on 21/6/13, approx. 10 months post-op. Note the surgeon's pen markings. They will draw marks to ensure the right bits are taken off, or put in, as in my case.

During the first day after the operation, I was given six hourly antibiotics intravenously and a painkiller underneath my tongue. To assist with stopping the formation of blood clots I was also given Heparin injections three times a day. My stomach became quite bruised and tender by the time I left the hospital. Some journal entries from the days in the hospital.

Saturday 12th April: *"Stiff in the chest both sides but ok. Ladies in the ward (I later referred to them as my friends), Joan-across from me, Ida next to her, Hillary next to me."*

Sunday 13th April: *"Have a large Seroma near left side armpit. Also Haematoma on left side mastectomy. The doctor will keep an eye on both. Going for little walks every day. Still doing gentle exercises and shoulder rolls. Sunday night: Didn't sleep well at all. Cannula vein in my hand 'tissued' this morning. Very painful when trying to push antibiotics through. Felt like a pin cushion. Had two nurses and three doctors trying to find another vein. Was very hard and very painful. Doc finally found a small one at ten pm."*

A Seroma is a pocket of clear serous fluid that sometimes develops in the body after surgery.

A Haematoma is a solid swelling of clotted blood within the tissues.

A Tissued vein occurs when a cannula is dislodged from a vein or there is leakage between the cannula and the wall of the vein.

Monday 14th April: *"Left hand and wrist swollen and sore. Very tired and my arm very sore. Having no problems from the chest. Doc says Seroma has gone down a bit, so keep an eye on it. Monday night, cannula vein tissued again. Not happy now. Didn't sleep much at all. Worried about another cannula. Want oral antibiotics instead."*

Tuesday 15th April: *"Really tired. Was so happy doc decided to give oral antibiotics yay! Really relieved. Arm is so sore. Pathology girls having trouble finding veins for a blood test. Took 3 girls to find one. DON'T LIKE NEEDLES ANYMORE!!! Gentle shoulder rolls and chicken wing exercises. Doesn't hurt at all really. Had one drain taken out today. Right side. Good to have one out. Quite surprised how easy it is to move my left arm after mastectomy. Seroma a bit smaller. L/S chest quite lumpy with the expander. Can feel it and see it. R/S looks and feels good."*

Wednesday 16th April: *"Had rounds at ten am. Doc said have to check with Dr. Ponniah re-drains. At two pm was told both drains can come out and go home!!! 1 drain came out okay-painful but okay. Other drain VERY VERY HARD AND PAINFUL. The nurse tried to take out drain by pulling gently but was really painful. She went and got a doctor who kept trying. OMG-so painful. Was crying and just wanted it all to be over. Doc wanted to give painkiller but I said by the time that works, it'll be over. Every time I breathed, he pulled. So painful. Took about twenty mins all up. Very shocked and crying so was my poor baby who held my hand the whole time. The tissue had started to clot around the drain holes which made it really hard to remove. My babe and I were both having a good cry after. It wasn't very nice. Hope it doesn't happen next time. Left hos at three-thirty pm. Had a quick cuppa. Very sore bruised arm. Sore tummy. Chest doesn't feel too bad."*

Wednesday afternoon/evening: *"Finally*

at home. Very emotional. Keep crying. Walked around the house a bit and then went straight to bed. My babe and I both slept quite well. Bit uncomfortable until I got the pillows right. Taking 6 hourly antibiotics and Panadol every 4 hours. Doing exercises regularly. Quite easy to do them. Shoulder rolling gently often."

Thursday 17th April: *"Little bit tired. Had arvo sleep. Bed at 11 pm. Slept through till 4.30am. Longest sleep yet. Bit stiff over chest and back."*

Friday 18th April: *"Up at four-thirty am. Couldn't sleep. Took Panadol and got up and had a banana and milo and wrote in journal. Felt a bit red and rashy on chest last night. Keep an eye on it. Good Friday today. Feeling tightness around drain sites on both sides. Might start gentle massage over bandages. (On How am I feeling scale?- 4- good)."*

Saturday 19th April: *"Expander in right side looks and feels good. Quite firm to touch. Left side- oh dear! Still, have haematoma near the top of armpit and centre of chest and sore under left chest near drain sites."*

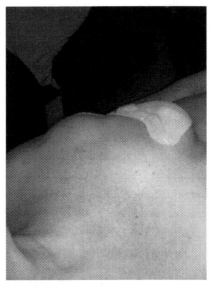

Top right of the picture where the doctor has drawn
the arrow, you can see the bulge from the haematoma.

After I left the hospital on the 16th April, I
was given a post-op appointment date for the 24th
of April. During the appointment, Dr. Ponniah
asked me to remove my shirt so she could examine
the wound site and remove the outer bandages.
After examining the site, she told me there were a
lot of blood clots under the expander and near the
armpit, so we would wait and see how the healing
went before doing anything more. She removed
the outer bandages and 3 days later I removed the

steri-strips that had covered the wounds, which had been glued closed. (Pictured below)

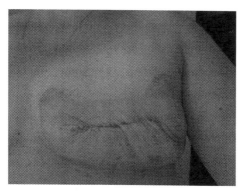

Left-hand side Mastectomy. Thirteen days post op. Expanders have one hundred ml in volume so far. Breast tissue removed weighed seven hundred gms approx.

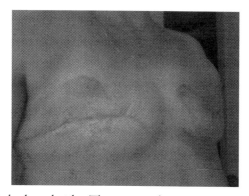

Right-hand side. The original mastectomy scar starts from the middle of my chest and curves along to about half of the scar that now appears.

A journal entry from 27th April: *"Left side still very tender and lumpy to see and touch. Right side really good. Feeling better. Chest sometimes feels really tight on both sides as though it is being squeezed. Take Panadol when I need to. Antibiotics finished last night yay! Still gently doing chicken wing exercises, physio says that's good for now. Not sleeping to bad. Had 3 big hot flushes which woke me up. Back to work tomorrow. Must remember to take it easy. Not driving yet. Catch the bus to work. (3 weeks) Still need an afternoon nap. Will come home from work and have a nap."*

At my post op appointment, the doctor had made an appointment to see me again to check on the healing of the haematoma. She had said that if the left side was not swollen, she could do the second expansion. So on the 22nd May, I saw Dr. Ponniah again so she could inspect her work. After doing an examination of the left side chest wall, my doctor suggested that I have an ultrasound done. The ultrasound would show anything abnormal and also any clots etc. So due to the pain I still had particularly on the left side and the swelling that was still present, no expansion was done to either expander. I was a bit disappointed, but as I was still in some degree of discomfort, I tried not to become despondent. Dr. Ponniah said she would put in a request for the ultrasound and I would get the appointment sent in the mail. Before I left, another appointment was made for me to attend the clinic again in about four weeks. I left the doctor's office and was seen by the physio. The physio checked my scars and the movement of my arms. She recommended that I stay doing the basic exercises, lifting my elbows towards the ceiling and out to the sides. This was enough for now she said, as she didn't want me to overdo it.

An appointment was made for the 9th June for the ultrasound and I went along hopeful that this would end my wait to have another expansion. The results showed that there was a slight curl in the top of the left side expander and also showed clotting and swelling near the left armpit. These results would be sent to my doctor.

It was good to be back at work during this time, as work helped to occupy my mind. Peng and I always had a laugh and our customers were always happy, as they were going on holidays, so my environment was very positive. During this time, I went braless. I now wore plain cotton crop tops. I didn't want to aggravate my swellings and

I felt comfortable, albeit a bit flat chested. The expanders made my chest look a bit square, so it wasn't the most attractive look, but it was the means to an end.

On the 19th June, I attended the breast clinic hopeful for an expansion. Once inside the doctor's office, Dr. Ponniah checked my right and left sides and declared that it was expansion time! I was so excited.

There is a process involved when doing an expansion. Firstly, the doctor finds the port at the top of the expander which can usually be felt just underneath the skin. This is where the needle will be inserted. After sterilizing the area well, a syringe filled with the required volume of saline solution is then slowly pushed into the expander. During the process, I felt the area tighten as the volume of the expanders increased, and my skin was slowly stretched again. I was not scared about this process and it took only about twenty minutes. I didn't feel any pain or need an anaesthetic. I think this is because the skin on my chest was quite numb. To this day, almost five years later, the sensation is still numb, over most of the surface area of both breasts.

I left the doctor's office happy, knowing the

process had gone a bit further that day. The process of expansion can be completed in as little as six weeks depending on the doctor and the patient. I was hoping to be filled to the volume that Dr. Ponniah had suggested, of four hundred mills each side, within four months. Which meant having an expansion every month. Well, we were a little bit behind already, but all going well, I was hoping for another expansion in a month's time.

So, I now had two hundred mills, in both expanders. After a week or so though, I noticed that the left side seemed a bit bigger, but the right side didn't seem to be getting as big. I decided I would keep an eye on this myself. I asked Martin a couple of times, what he thought. He couldn't really see any big differences, so I thought maybe it's just me.

On the 10th of July, I went again for another expansion. As the surgeons are very busy and also need a holiday, for this visit, I did not see Dr. Ponniah. I saw a very nice surgeon though, who performed another expansion of one hundred mills, which went very smoothly. I did discuss with him, my opinion that I didn't feel the right side was expanding at the same rate as the left side. He told me not to worry, and that at the next expansion, hopefully, a difference could be seen if there was any problem. After another week, I really knew something was up. The right side was definitely smaller and Martin could also tell by this stage.

Martin came along to the next visit to the clinic for an expansion on the 5th August. At this appointment, I saw Dr. Ponniah and also her colleague that I had seen at the previous appointment. I voiced my concerns and Dr. Ponniah agreed I was probably right. She suggested we do another expansion that day and then asked me to come back again in two weeks. She would see if the expansion of the right side had been successful.

I returned to the clinic on the 19th August, somewhat disheartened. I knew it was just one of those things that can happen. It was nobody's fault. After Dr. Ponniah examined me, she said the right side expander would definitely have to be replaced! Bummer. As I was in the public health system, I didn't know how long I would have to wait for this operation. It had been about five months since the operation to insert the expanders. I had thought the expansion would be done by now, and instead, I was going to have another operation. Dr. Ponniah said she would do her best to fit me in when she could. I was happy at least to know that she was doing her best to help me. I feel this helped me to stay positive. Knowing that she cared and felt for our situation. So I left her office that day, wondering when the operation would be, and going back into waiting mode.

About a week later, I received an appointment letter for my pre-admission which was on the 22nd of September. A surgery date of the 2nd October was given for the replacement of the expander. I would only have to stay overnight which I was very happy about.

The surgery went really well and I had two hundred millilitres put into the expander straight away, as the skin had already been expanded. I was allowed home the next morning after being seen by the doctors on rounds, with some oral antibiotics to take for a week or so. I could tell after a day or so that the volume in the new expander was bigger than the last one I had. Needless to say, I was really happy with the outcome and the great work performed by my lovely surgeon. She also used the same scar as before, so I didn't have another one, which was very good (see below).

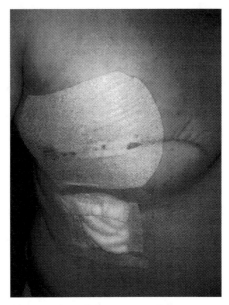

The top bandage covers the incision
wound and the lower bandage is covering
where the drain tube was removed.

I had a post op appointment on the 23rd of
October. Unfortunately, Dr. Ponniah said I had
to wait for another six to eight weeks before
another expansion could be done. This was to
give the surgery scar, more time to heal before
it was stretched again. I understood what I was
told, and wanted everything done well, so I went
home unexpanded!

Finally, on the 6th of November, I was able to
have the second expansion of one hundred mills,

which now took the volume to three hundred mills. I was chafing at the bit now, so Dr. Ponniah said I could come back in two weeks for the third expansion. Yay!!!

Following this, on the 4th December 2014, I had the final expansion to the right side of one hundred mills. Five hundred mills finally. We had reached the end, thank goodness. Dr. Ponniah decided to add a further fifty mills to the left side and had increased the volume on the right side. This was to compensate for the decreased fat in the right side compared to the left. Dr. Ponniah and I were both really happy. I could tell she was happy for me too. Now we would begin another waiting game. Again, my doctor said she would do her best to have my surgery completed as soon as possible. It had been nearly nine months since the second mastectomy and expander insertion. Time flies. I left the doctor's office and said that I hoped I would see her sooner rather than later.

Over the next twenty months, I had surgery scheduled and then cancelled, twice. I found during that time, that the expanders seemed to have moved to quite a high position on my chest. I made mention to Martin many times, that I hoped when the implants were put in, they didn't fit in where the expanders had been! The expanders had been in since 11th April 2014.

We had continued to get on with our lives during this time and had decided that life was meant to be lived now. Not when we got older. My dream had always been to travel to the Greek island of Santorini. My wonderful husband said to me, we should just do it! So I did what I do best, I organised and planned. We saved and saved and had the holiday of a lifetime booked from the 13th – 29th March 2016.

Funnily enough, I received an appointment letter to visit the breast clinic at the end of February 2016. I was so happy and relieved that something might get done. I attended the clinic and was excited to see my wonderful Dr. Ponniah again. I was just about jumping out of my skin, especially when the doctor asked me if I would be available to have my surgery to replace the expanders with implants on the 1st April 2016! What.?!

Now I do understand what you are probably thinking however, it is the truth! Needless to say, I was one happy camper. Dr. Ponniah organised the paperwork and we went through it again, as we had done so many times before. We told the doctor about our upcoming trip and how amazing we thought it was going to be. But to top it off with an operation to finally get my implants, was more than I could have asked for! We knew that when we came home from our holiday that we would have a couple of days to get acclimated before having the surgery, so we left the clinic appointment with nothing but positive energy. I was so happy.

We left for my dream holiday and it was all I could have asked for and more. Martin and I were so thankful to be there. I was so grateful to be alive. Even though we were so happy, we did cry a lot on that holiday. The views that we saw around every corner, could only have been created by the God that had allowed me to live; they were breathtaking. Martin and I had trouble believing we were actually standing on the Island of Santorini, looking out over the Caldera with the bluest skies that you have ever seen above us. Every time we got overwhelmed, which was a lot, the tears ran.

As this was our first overseas holiday together and my lovely mum had offered to care for the children, we wanted to check in every couple of days to see that everyone was okay. On one particular phone call, my son Tyson said he had taken a phone call from someone from the hospital. Immediately my heart went to my mouth. I asked Tyson what they had said, but he couldn't recall clearly what had been discussed. Just something about my appointment. Huh! I don't think Tyson knew how important that phone call was to me, so I took matters into my own hand and called the hospital myself, after getting off the phone with the kids.

Upon ringing the hospital and being put in touch with the booking clerk, I found out that my appointment had been brought forward to the 31st of March. Oh my god, how amazing. I thanked the clerk and hung up the phone and Martin and I sat in disbelief. This was getting better. Now when we arrived home, we had two days before my surgery. Luckily for us, there was a fantastic laundry on Santorini, so the day before we left, we took all our dirty clothes to be washed for fifteen euros! We collected our washing which was washed and folded and packed in two neat bags. I was happy that we didn't have that job to do when we arrived home.

On the 31st March 2016, we went to the hospital at 6.30am. After such a long time having the expanders in, I was so ready to have them gone, and replaced with my new boobies. It had been just under two years since the second mastectomy and insertion of the expanders. Although they serve a great purpose, stretching the skin ready for the implants, they are not the best-looking things in the world. For nearly two years I had not been able to wear nice little tops, as everything looked odd and square. It did play havoc with my self-esteem and how I viewed myself. But that was all going to change in just under five hours.

The surgery was successful, starting at eight thirty am and finishing at eleven thirty am. After spending an hour or so in recovery, I was taken up to a medical ward by one thirty pm. I would spend a couple of days in hospital until the drainage volume was acceptable. I had two drains, one on each side, just under the chest area.

A journal entry for 31ˢᵗ March: *"No sleep for two nights. Doctors busy with the lady in next bed. Very tired. Up Friday morning at seven and walked to get a cuppa. Nurses very happy!"*

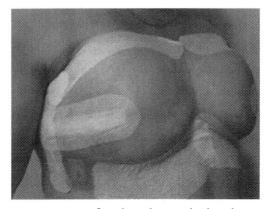

The tape on top of and underneath the chest area helps to stabilise the implants. The middle piece hides the surgery scar and the small rectangle is the drain site. It would stay like this until the post-op appointment. The Velcro Binder was worn around my chest and sat on top of the top bandage.

The day following my surgery, Martin came in to visit and as always had little treats for me. One of these little treats was a photo album he had hurriedly put together, with some of the highlights of our Grecian holiday. We sat together on my hospital bed and looked through the small album, remembering our wonderful holiday. What a lucky girl I am, to have a husband like this. He always thinks of the little things. Love you baby.

On Saturday the 2nd April, the doctors came

to do their rounds in the ward about ten thirty am. Dr. Ponniah was happy with the drainage volumes so I was allowed to go home. Yay. The drains came out well with no issues at all. Martin came in and had brought the Velcro breast binder that Dr. Ponniah has asked us to buy when we had our last appointment. This elastic binder is worn around the top of the implants and secured with Velcro to assist with keeping the implants stable and to offer a degree of compression. I would be wearing the band for two weeks, as well as the post-surgery bra. We headed off for home mid-morning.

A journal entry for 2nd – 5th April: *"Doing gentle chicken wing exercises every day. Wearing Velcro band across the top of the chest. All going well. Left one still bigger than the right one."*

On the 15th of April, I had my post op appointment. After I removed the Velcro band, Dr. Ponniah took off the bandaging. I voiced my concerns about the difference in size between the right and left sides. And also how high the implants were sitting on my chest. Dr. Ponniah explained that the top of the left chest was still swollen. She said we would have another appointment in two to three months and if there was still a vast difference in size, she could do some fat removal from around the bottom and side of the breast. I felt relieved and happy that my concerns were being validated. I always felt that Dr. Ponniah listened to me and I never felt anything other than fully supported by her and her team. She also said that soon after the next appointment, we could discuss nipple reconstruction.

As with the choice to either have an immediate reconstruction or a delayed one or to even have one at all, the choice to have a nipple reconstruction or not is also available. I have heard of many women choosing to have three-dimensional tattooing of their nipples, and the pictures I have seen are awesome. For me though, I needed the nipple to be tactile. I wanted to feel something there in the place that I had felt something for the past forty-eight years. Until that appointment though, it was back to work. I had changed my employment since 2013 and now had an admin role in a confectionery wholesaler, so under strict instructions by my doctor not to do any heavy lifting of stock etc., I went back to work until the post-op appointment which would be on the 22nd July 2016.

As the days and then weeks and then months

went by after the operation, I didn't get any happier. This was due to the fact that the implants had moved to the exact position that the expanders had been in for the past two years. I kept saying to Martin "See, I told you this would happen." Martin could tell I was unhappy. I just hated to look at my chest in the mirror. My chest didn't look any better in clothing either. I was so upset, as I had waited so long for this to happen and it looked awful.

Finally, the 22nd of July came around, so Martin and I went to the appointment at the hospital. I usually bounced through the door but I didn't feel very bouncy that day. Dr. Ponniah asked me to undress the top half behind the curtain and then asked if she could examine my chest. She felt around and looked at both sides of my chest, and then declared that I had Capsular Contracture. I would need revision surgery. I cried.

First time ever, in the clinic. I told Dr. Ponniah that I was so disappointed and my chest looked awful. She said she was disappointed too, but it happened sometimes.

She said, "Don't worry, we'll fix them!"

She then proceeded to tell us of a conference that she had been to recently. She said while she was at the conference she was thinking about my situation and the concerns I had voiced at our last meeting. Really! I was gobsmacked that my wonderful doctor had been thinking of little old me while she was at a conference. Dr. Ponniah asked me if she could try a procedure using a new implant called a teardrop shape and a product called Veritas mesh. This mesh would be attached to the pectoral muscle, which would extend it. In my case, the pectoral muscles were holding the implants too high. The use of the mesh would create a 'hammock' that would cradle the implant giving a more natural droop, shape and contour to the completed breast. The doctor said she would also do a slight fat reduction in the left side and she would also make the incision underneath the breast, so it wouldn't show.

I was over the moon. I couldn't wait. Talk about excited. I gave Dr. Ponniah a big hug. After getting dressed, the doctor looked in her calendar and asked "Would the 18th of August be okay?"

Ummm, yes. This was only four weeks away. My poor boss once again got a phone call asking "Please could I have more time off?" I have been blessed with wonderful bosses throughout this experience, that's for sure. Thankyou bosses!

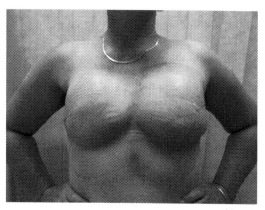

This photo was taken at the post-op appointment on July 22nd, 2016. Nearly four months since the implant exchange operation and you can see how high the implants were sitting. Also, note the size difference between the left and right sides.

Well, I was glad that the time went quickly, as I waited for the next operation. I was getting really excited. That excitement, however, was not to last. I received a call about a week and a half before the operation. The booking clerk told me that my operation had to be rescheduled for the 25th of August. I had to wait another week. Okay. It wasn't as bad as I had thought. I can do this.

I had my scheduled pre-admission appointment on the 11th of August. I was told that after the operation, I would be in the hospital again for about a six-day stay. I remembered to pack everything for this visit. Ear plugs, check. Eyeshade, check. Music, check.

Martin and I once again headed to the hospital on the surgery day, 25th August 2016. The surgery went really well. Journal entries during this stay: *"Had new implants and Veritas mesh which all worked really well. Yay. My boobies are beautiful!!! Came out of surgery in recovery and Dr. P (Ponniah) was really happy and said they looked awesome and took a photo to show me!! So funny, I couldn't see a thing cos I had no glasses on and also still half zonked. When finally in Day surgery ward, showed Martin and he cried. He said they looked just like normal boobs. I look at them a lot!!"*

I didn't get to a general medical ward on this stay, I had to stay in the day surgery ward. This was weird, as there were men and women in the ward. On every other visit I have had to stay in for, I have only ever had women in the ward. So this was something new. I had to stay in for six days, as the output volume of the drains was still high. I had really lovely nurses again during this stay. I was finally allowed to go home on the 31st August, which I was really happy about. The implants were totally different than the other set.

They were softer and lower and looked really good underneath my clothing. I was a happy girl.

Dr. Ponniah had arranged for my post-op appointment to be on the 9th of September. I arrived at the appointment with a huge smile on my face. My doctor explained about the capsular contracture. During the operation, she had taken out the implant and also the capsule of scar tissue surrounding it. The new teardrop shape implants and mesh were now positioned on my chest in a very natural way. We were both smiling at her handiwork. I couldn't thank her enough. She was so pleased, that she asked if I would allow the medical photographer to take some pictures of my new chest. I readily agreed and saw the photographer with a nurse a short while later. The doctor said she would try and organise an appointment to discuss the nipple reconstruction, as soon as possible.

I told her "We've come this far, a bit longer can't hurt."

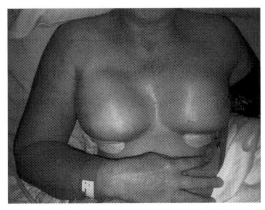

This picture was taken once I was back in the day of surgery ward. You can already see how different the implants are to the previous ones. These are more natural looking. Also, as the capsule of scar tissue was removed, they eventually found their own place to sit.

A bit longer ended up being the 9th of December 2016. I attended the appointment with Dr. Ponniah and she explained how she would form the new nipples. She would create a flap of skin at the site where the new nipple would be positioned, which would then be folded over and around itself and stitched into place. After the nipples healed, I could then get them tattooed and also the areola to complete my new breasts. I was once again in the very capable hands of my lovely surgeon. I trusted that she would do the very best she could to reproduce a pair of nipples for me. We completed all the necessary paperwork for the operation, so we were good to go, except we needed a date. As the surgery was elective, I would be on a waitlist until space became available in the surgeon's schedule. I received the waitlist paperwork and sent it back to the hospital around December 19th, 2016. And now we wait.

Martin and I once again got on with our lives. Back to work and also planning another holiday. This time we were off to Singapore in March 2017. We were very excited about going. I had visited this lovely country briefly for work back in 2000, and I told Martin I remembered how safe I felt and how clean the place was, so our decision was made. We booked our tickets and accommodation and were all set to go.

In early March I received a call from one of the breast centre nurses. She said Dr. Ponniah had asked if I would like to have my surgery on the 16th March 2017. I excitedly answered yes, and then asked if the doctor still remembered that we were going on holidays on the 25th March. We both agreed that she wouldn't have asked if it would have been a problem, so it was scheduled. I attended a pre-admission appointment on the 9th of March. This would be quite a quicker operation than the past ones and I would leave hospital on the same day. We were finally coming to the end of the road.

There was no way Martin was going to miss this last operation. So together again, off we went to the hospital. Once we arrived at the day of surgery ward and handed in our paperwork, we took a seat and got out our books to read. A short while later I was asked to follow a nurse to change into my lovely blue surgery gown and paper bikini. I was then shown to my bed and rugged up. With Martin by my side, the nurses and anaesthetists performed their duties in readiness for the operation.

About half an hour before the surgery, Dr. Ponniah and one of her colleagues asked me to follow them into a change room, as they had to draw some measurements on my chest. I followed them into the change room. What followed was one of the funniest times I have had throughout the whole experience.

There we were, three adult women, one with her gown around her waist (me, of course), and the other two drawing on her with a purple pen. There is a certain way of measuring to make sure the nipple is positioned accurately. The doctors also had some round electrode stickers which, by accident, I'm sure, quite closely resembled nipples. These were used to imitate the nipple to allow correct positioning. Ingenius!! We stuck two of them on my chest and then headed into a bathroom to use the mirror, so I could hold the gown up over my chest and see if the projection and placement of the 'nipple' were correct. We were all laughing and I kept saying how real they looked. I wanted to go and show Martin my 'new nipples'. What a fun time that was, but it did work. We made our way back into the change room and the doctors finished their measurements and drawings. Thank god for pre-planning! And for wonderful doctors with amazing bedside manners and beautiful souls. I was so blessed to have these ladies as my surgeons.

I made my way back to my bed and retold the story to Martin. He said the whole ward could hear us laughing in the bathroom and change room. It was a great end to a long journey. The operation was very successful, and I now had two little nipples. Later that afternoon, I was taken to the day surgery ward and kept under observation for a few more hours.

It was quite funny with this operation, as I hadn't asked what would happen after the surgery to the wound site. I just expected that I would be bandaged in some way, as I had been for every previous surgery. This was why it hadn't bothered me about having the surgery so close to our holiday departure.

When I became clearer in the head, Martin and I looked at my chest. I had what I thought looked like PopTop caps over these little buds. (See below) I had no pain at all.

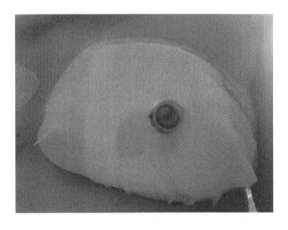

Later that evening, one of Dr. Ponniah's colleagues came to see me making sure everything was good, so we could go home. We discussed the fact that we were going to Singapore the following week. I was then told that I couldn't get my chest wet at all.

What!! No swimming or normal shower. That was a bummer. We had a rooftop pool at our apartment and had planned on swimming every day. The doctor also explained that I had vomited after the operation. I had been assessed by the anaesthetist but had to be aware of the risk of developing a chest infection. I was to have a post-op appointment on the 21st April.

"Wow," I said to the doctor, "That will be almost five weeks post-op, is that not too long?"

The doctor said she would double check with Dr. Ponniah and if anything changed she would call us. We left the hospital with wound care instructions and big smiley faces.

We were told by the nurses to check every few hours for blood flow, by using a cotton tip and gently pressing the tip of the nipple and watching to see the colour return. This would indicate good blood flow. We did this over the next few hours until bed and again in the morning.

As I had researched pretty much every aspect of my treatments, I had previously read that, as with any tissue transplant or reconstruction, there is always a chance that the tissue may become necrotic, due to inhibited blood flow to the area.

I had made a joke with my mum once and said "Great, I'll get new boobs, and then my nipples will fall off and die! I'll be walking along and trip on something, and someone will say, "Is that yours?" We laughed so hard at that. It seemed even more real now though.

By mid-afternoon on Sunday 17th however, I was getting quite worried about the dark black patch I could see on the left nipple. Without hesitation, Martin drove me to S.C.G.H where we attended the emergency department. We were seen by a doctor and related our story to him. I was asked to wait in a room and a short while later he handed me a telephone and said that Dr. Ponniah was on the line. I spoke to my doctor for a short while and then gave the phone back to the emergency doctor. My doctor stated that everything was probably fine and that there wouldn't be much she could do if the tissue had started to feel the effects of limited blood flow. We had to hope for the best. I thanked her for talking to me and apologised for taking her time on the weekend. Martin and I thanked the emergency doctor and made our way home. I was hoping and praying that my nipples would both survive.

About five thirty pm I was resting on my bed, reading a book when my mobile phone rang. I didn't recognise the number but decided to answer it anyway.

"Hello," I said.

"Hello, Caroline, this is your surgeon Dr. Ponniah," came the reply.

Oh my god, really, now my surgeon is doing house calls! Talk about above and beyond. I was gobsmacked but worried all at the same time. My doctor explained to me that she hadn't fully realised how close my holidays were to the surgery. There was a slight misunderstanding in the timing of it all. She said that there was no way she could wait until the 21st April to see me. The new post-op date would be the 10th April.

"I want to see you tomorrow (Monday) and also Friday if that's possible. I will change the dressings and show you how to change them if you need to, while you are away. Is that going to be okay with you?" Dr. Ponniah asked.

I told my doctor that would be totally fine and that I was feeling much better now that I would be seeing her sooner than the 21st. I visited the breast clinic on both days. On the Friday visit, my doctor arranged a small bag of dressings that I would take with me on holidays, in case I needed to change them. She also said to me that if I had any concerns while we were away, that I could call her or send her a photo, and she would tell me what to do.

I said to her "There are hospitals in Singapore!"

She said it was up to me, but that she would be more than happy to help if we needed it. Blessed am I. The funny thing was, our apartment in Singapore was just around the corner from a rather large hospital. Doubly blessed.

Well, we headed off on Saturday 25th March 2017 to sunny, humid Singapore. Because I had two little pop top caps sticking out from my chest, we had devised a way to make them less conspicuous. I did not want anyone thinking I was Madonna Mk2. We bought some nursing pads and I cut large round circles and then one smaller one in the middle like a doughnut. We then stuck these around the existing dressing to 'fill in' the height difference. I couldn't wear little shoestring tops, but at least my flowing tops were acceptable and covered everything. They were extremely hot though, being polyester.

The first day in Singapore was hot and sticky. We headed up to the rooftop pool. I was carefully able to sit on the side of the pool while Martin bobbed around under the lukewarm water. He is so considerate, that he only went swimming that once. We tended to rest in our air-conditioned apartment instead. Showering was torture. I had bought some waterproof dressing covers, which of course didn't work. I was lucky enough though, that the shower had a hand held shower head. I would get in the shower and turn on the water. Carefully wet my legs and stomach. Lean over and wet my arms and then wet a flannel for my face. Lastly, my back got a quick wash. Arghhh. I had two weeks of this. We also had to be careful when we were out and about as there are a lot of people in Singapore in a very small area. I tended to walk behind Martin so I didn't get my chest knocked, particularly on the train. Anyway, our first time in Singapore was great, albeit a bit hot, sticky and uncomfortable without a proper swim or shower. My nipples stood up to the challenge beautifully with no problems at all. Thanks to my wonderful surgeon.

I attended my appointment on the 10th of April at the breast clinic. I had bought a Ferrero Rocher chocolate flower bouquet from a wonderful store called Edible Blooms. I didn't know how else to thank my surgeon for all her amazing work over the past five years. I soon found out that my doctor couldn't be there that day, so I saw one of her colleagues instead. I had seen him before. He carefully removed all the dressings and asked if I had had any issues. I told him that everything had gone well and I was just looking forward to having a proper shower. He said that Dr. Ponniah would like to see me again on the 21st of April, so she could see the nipples for herself. I said I thought I should bring the chocolates back on the next visit, and he thought that was very wise too!

That night I had the best shower I think I have ever had. I had to be extremely careful with my new nipples as they were still healing. I could see little bits of stitches sticking out the tops and sides which was really funny looking. They looked really good. I knew that after some time the size of them would reduce once they had healed fully. I knew my doctor was going to be pleased.

I went to the hospital on the 21st of April, for what was to be the last time. My doctor called my name and I went forward with the chocolate bouquet and gave it to her and added a little hug.

I also included a card where we thanked her for all her care and attention over the past years, as well as that of her staff. I really feel their care made such a huge impact on my recovery. We checked out my new nipples and I could tell she was very pleased with her work.

After a little chat, my doctor said that I could now be discharged as a patient. Wow! I said my tear-filled goodbyes and there were thank yous and hugs. As I made my way down the corridor of the breast clinic, I was happy thinking to myself that this experience was now finally over. I called Martin once I was sitting in my car, and told him I had been discharged. He asked me how I felt about that, and I cried and said I was so thankful it was over and that I was still here. He agreed with me!

Martin's perspective on Reconstruction

I believed that this was going to be the easiest part of the whole journey. Remove the breast, stick in some expanders, fill them up, whack in a couple of implants and there you have it, new boobs. Boy was I wrong.

The hardest thing about reconstruction was the waiting. The Breast Centre is a very busy place. Every time we went there it was packed. The other thing was, Caroline no longer had cancer, so really the priority was to help those that needed attention to save their life. The staff at the Breast Centre were amazing and nothing seemed too much bother for them. They were always happy and attentive to the patient's needs.

But, as they were so busy and the priority was given to patients with cancer, it did mean some long waits between various operations. Caroline has mentioned the dates while writing. This is something that could happen and you need to be prepared for it. Obviously, some of the problems that we encountered, did slow the whole process down a bit.

In a selfish way, this was hard for me. Why should we have to wait? I wanted my wife to have her reconstruction finished so that she could feel, for lack of a better word, normal again. She had been through so much and been so patient. But, as I said, the breast centre is a very busy place and this was not about me but about lots of people going through the same thing we were.

The other thing that was hard to deal with, was watching my beautiful wife struggle with how she looked during this time. One breast, then flat breasts, then one breast (expander) again, then a set of breasts on her shoulders (maybe an exaggeration) and finally a set that has made her (and me) happy.

Caroline mentioned earlier, that I had said to her that I didn't have a preference for the type of implants that she chose. Well, maybe not entirely true. When she said she wanted the round and perky set, I was a bit concerned that they wouldn't suit her body. I believed that the teardrop-shaped would be a better fit. But would I say that to her? NO. These were a part of her that she would have to live with for a very long time, so in my opinion, the choice was entirely hers. As long as she was happy I was happy. This was the set that she had to have removed and she chose the teardrop set this time.

Having to deal with the stress of so many operations was hard for me to cope with. As mentioned earlier, I did stress quite a bit leading up to and during each operation. I always made sure I was there when Caroline went in for the operation and when she came out. We decided that for one of the operations I would go home (I am not sure why we did this. I think the operation was very late in the day so would have made a very long day for me to wait) and call to find out how it had gone. I vowed never to do this again, as I needed to see her and know she was alright. Maybe a bit of OCD but if that is what I needed to do to get through, then so be it.

When we look through photos that have been taken over the last 5 years, we can see the evidence of the various stages of Caroline's treatment and reconstruction. Pictures that have been taken of her in this time, are a constant reminder to both of us how parts of her have changed with chemotherapy and the operations. It is something to be aware of, as it is a constant reminder of what you have been through. I also think that it is an important thing for me to have as a reminder of what has happened, as I haven't had to live with all of the changes, pain, worry, and self-image, as nothing happened to my body. My beautiful wife has always been beautiful to me and still is. I am sure that I didn't even notice most of the time. I still had her and that is all that was important to me.

There is one particular photo of her on the Greek Island of Santorini (see below) where she is standing with the Caldera behind her. All she sees in that photo is her (in her words) square boobs (at this stage she had had her expanders and they had been filled). All I see is an amazing woman who has defeated this crappy disease, while keeping her sense of humour, compassion, empathy, love and her positive outlook to fulfill her dream of going to Santorini. The bonus in all of this, is that I got to go with her.

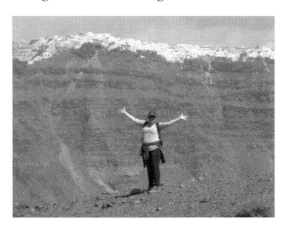

Caroline mentioned our holiday to Singapore after her nipple reconstruction. We did hesitate quite a bit during the whole five years, on when we should book anything like holidays, just in case an operation came up. Well, I am glad we did what we did and just booked. You have to live your life and take a couple of risks. The worse thing that could have happened is that we would have had to change the dates of our holiday. Would rather this, than wait around and not do anything just in case.

I tried to attend as many appointments with Caroline as I could but this was not always possible. As you may have gathered, we are very close and very supportive of each other. When I could not attend appointments with her, I insisted that she call me after and tell me everything that had happened and was discussed. I know this did not make up for not going with her but circumstances sometimes meant that I couldn't attend. I am sure she understood.

Chapter 4

Re-Building

Following the final operation in 2017 to have my nipples reconstructed, I was formally discharged about eight weeks later as an outpatient. With many tears, hugs and well wishes, I walked out of the breast clinic, after nearly five years. As I was making my way out, I was thinking this is it. No more operations, no more doctor's appointments, and as I had breast implants, no more breast checks.

I called Martin and told him I had been discharged and he asked me how I felt. I had heard that sometimes if the journey is particularly long, people can sometimes feel a bit lost as there are no more appointments or treatments to attend. I told Martin that I felt a sense of relief more than anything else. I was overjoyed beyond belief to be alive and by all accounts cancer free. I drove away from Sir Charles Gairdner Hospital smiling happily to myself and singing along to the radio.

We had finished with the hospital visits and doctor's appointments. Yet what people who haven't experienced this type of disease and treatment regime can't recognise, is the rebuilding that needs to occur for you and your family, in order to continue to live a long and happy life. This journey takes its toll. On the outside, I have new breasts, perky breasts, enviable breasts. On the inside, however, I have a conscious constant dread of this insipid disease returning, either to some other small part of my breasts that remain, or another organ of my body.

I hope this feeling will not always be conscious, as every sore joint and tired muscle has me thinking "Oh God please don't let it be anything." I can only trust in the process, as I trusted in the beginning, that I am now, where I am meant to be. I will say, however, that Breast Cancer Care W.A. do have psychologists available free of charge for families just like mine to talk with. I have said to Martin previously that I'll know when the time comes if I need to talk to someone and I've asked the same from him.

I actually had another two 'scares' in May/ June 2018. Five weeks after assisting an elderly lady who had fallen down backward on a moving travellator, I took myself off to the doctors. I was still in incredible pain by the end of every day and had trouble sitting down as well. I had tried to assist the lady as she fell, by scooping her up in my arms, forgetting of course that the travellator was still in motion and hastening me forward to a bad ending. I was then knocked back down onto my backside and upon trying to stand up after we had both caught our breath, had a very painful reminder of what had just happened.

The doctor asked of course why it had taken me five weeks to arrive at the surgery. I told her that as I had Rheumatoid Arthritis, I believed that all I was suffering with was deep tissue bruising. After examining me, she told me that she would like me to have an x-ray. She suspected that I had possibly injured my coccyx, which may account for the continued pain. I readily agreed as I was getting a bit tired of the pain.

I was able to have the x-ray that afternoon and the results were then sent back to the doctor. I received a call from the doctor the following day, asking me to come and see her again. I visited her the next morning and she gave me the results. She told me that the Radiologist was worried about a hazy white patch that was visible on my pelvis, on the x-ray. OMG! My stomach did a big flip I can tell you. The radiologist was suggesting that I have a bone scan to show a clearer picture of what the white patch may be.

"Okay," I said, "I'll get it organised."

Thankfully Medicare covered the cost of the bone scan which I had a few days later. A small dose of radiative liquid was injected into my vein, which over a two hour period circulated throughout my body. It then showed up areas that might be problematic such as tumours or fractures. The procedure did not hurt at all, only the insertion of the cannula into my crusty hard veins in my left arm, a sad reminder of the chemotherapy treatment. There was also a CT scan done. The results were once again sent to the doctor.

I visited her again a week later. She gave me the great news that there was no tumour present. The radiologists couldn't explain the white patch on the x-ray. I'll take that. I did, however, have a fractured coccyx. That, I can live with.

At the end of this appointment, the doctor

asked me when I had last had a mammogram or ultrasound performed on my breasts. I told her that I had not had anything of the sort since the last implant operation in late 2016. However, I told her that every year when I have my pap smear done, my regular doctor always does a breast examination. As this doctor hadn't seen my breasts before she asked if she could perform a manual breast exam. I told her that was fine and popped up on the bed. As she performed the check she got to a spot at the right side of my breast and asked if the little nodule she could feel was normal. I felt it myself and said, "Well I'm not sure." She wasn't happy about that answer and due to my history, recommended that I have an ultrasound as soon as possible. As I'm not one to leave things, I made an appointment for the following week and off I went.

As the technician was performing the ultrasound she came across the same place as the doctor had and scanned it for a short while. She completed the scan and then told me she would have the senior technician look over the scan. When she returned a short while later, she told me that the senior technician suggested that a biopsy be taken of the nodule to determine exactly what it was. It could be scar tissue, a fatty deposit or something far worse. The technician said the results of the scan would be sent to my doctor to determine where the biopsy would take place.

I returned again the next day to see my doctor. She proposed calling my surgeon from S.C.G.H to discuss how to continue with the treatment. After talking to my surgeon and discussing the proposal with me at the same time, it was decided that I would return to S.C.G.H and attend the breast clinic for an examination and possible biopsy. I would receive the appointment time and date in the mail.

I left the surgery and called Martin who hurriedly said: "Where's a bucket?"

Poor baby. We had a laugh over the phone even though we knew we were both freaking out just a little bit!

I received the appointment letter about two weeks later and attended the breast clinic as requested. On entering the clinic room the ladies behind the counter recognised me and greeted me warmly. I was given my coloured card and went into the waiting room.

My name was called by my lovely surgeon Dr. Ponniah a short while later. We had a brief chat about how I'd been and the ultrasound results and then she performed a manual examination. She could also feel the nodule and then asked me if I had time to have the biopsy performed that day.

"I sure do," was my reply. I was told I would also be having a mammogram.

Doctor Ponniah then noticed that I had been on Tamoxifen for nearly five years. I told her I had one month to go. She asked me if I would like to stay on Tamoxifen for another five years. I said that I had read about studies for and against taking it for an extra five years and what the studies had concluded. However, I told her that regardless of what the studies showed, I would love to take it for another five years. Again for me, it's a small price to pay, for some extra piece of mind and I'm sure she could see that also. I thanked my lovely doctor again and headed off with a breast care nurse.

The nurse who took me through to another waiting room where ladies were all waiting to have their ultrasounds, mammograms, and biopsies performed. I was called in for my mammogram about ten minutes later.

As I was being put into position for the

mammogram, I told the technician that as I had implants I didn't think a mammogram could be performed. She explained to me that they had been advised it was safe to perform a mammogram on implants as long as the correct pressure was applied. Well, that was news to me.

The mammogram took about fifteen minutes to perform. The technician took quite a few pictures as it was a difficult position to scan, being on the right side nearly underneath my armpit. She eventually got the pictures she needed and I went back out to the waiting room.

As I was waiting, I looked around at the other ladies seated around the room and wondered how they were all coping with whatever news they had received or were still waiting for. This disease touches so many lives. Even if a cancer diagnosis is not given, the stress and discomfort the experience causes can still leave a lasting impression. I felt for every last one of them.

I was called into a clinic room to have the biopsy done. I would be having a Fine needle aspiration to determine whether or not cancer cells were present in the nodule. As I had previously had an FNA performed, I knew exactly what to expect and so as the technician performed the procedure, we chatted about different things and it was all over in about thirty minutes. I was told by the technician that the results would be sent to my doctor. However, my surgeon said that the breast clinic nurses would call me with the results as well. Thank god we wouldn't have to wait long for the results.

Martin and I had organised to go to Albany for the long weekend in June to stay with relatives. About two days before we were due to go, I received a call from the breast care nurses at S.C.G.H.

"The biopsy was clear and showed no cancer cells present. The nodule is possibly scar tissue or just fat cells," I was told by the nurse.

"Oh thank goodness, that's excellent news."

I jumped straight on the phone to Martin and told him our good news. He was just as relieved as I was. I did shed a few tears I will admit. The saying goes that 'Time heals all wounds.' Well, I hope in our case, that the wounds will gradually turn into scars that maybe won't disappear altogether, but will hopefully at least fade.

The different treatments I had, also took their own individual tolls on my body, mind, and spirit. Martin and I have had to change the way we look at different aspects of our personal lives, often on a very intimate level. We have had tears and triumphs and because we wanted our marriage to survive, we have tried to keep the lines of communication open with each other.

After the first mastectomy, my self-esteem took a battering. My thoughts weren't on how others would see me, but primarily how Martin would see me and how I saw myself. I had heard of other husbands not be able to cope and leaving the marriage. I certainly did not want that happening to mine. So we tried to be as honest as we could.

Earlier I related the incident about the first time Martin saw the first mastectomy scar, about four days after the operation. Well, even though he saw the scar that day, I still couldn't sleep without my PJ top on. I didn't take it off except to shower. I think it took about four to six weeks until I felt more comfortable to sleep without it on. I had to try and tell Martin that I knew he loved me, but it was how I was seeing my body that made me feel the way I was. I certainly did not feel attractive. Martin did his best to make sure I knew he still loved me.

He used to tell me "It's YOU that I love, not your boobs!"

Over time though, I have found that my breasts played a bigger part in lovemaking than I had thought. It was only now that I was minus one, that I began to see how much I missed it! As the surgery scar and surrounding tissue were quite tender for many months, touching of the other breast was done very carefully. I knew Martin didn't want to hurt me at all, so we always ventured to the 'other side' with trepidation. There were many times where either one of us would break down crying during these times, as the scar was a constant reminder of where we had just been. I believe we were still in shock from the whole experience. Just a small thing like a breast was affecting our lives intimately.

As I slept on our bed usually on my right side facing Martin, the lack of breast tissue was quite weird, once I was sleeping without my top on. I used to have a nice cushion to lean on, now there was nothing. I often used to wake up in the weeks following the op, and see Martin just looking at the scar. More often than not, he'd have a little cry and say "My poor baby."

The Cording that had developed along the inside of my right arm, as a result of the operation, also caused me a lot of pain and frustration. We had to do a lot of gentle massaging of the area under and along my arm, but also around the side of my chest. As the massage worked better when Martin could do it, we spent a short time every day for a long while, with some moisturiser and trying to ease the tightness of the cords. I felt very frustrated sometimes as the cords often used to grab at my arm and cause me to cry out with pain when I was doing things around the house or at work. While at work sometimes to ease the pain, I would hold my arm up against the wall where I used to sit and try and massage it when I had spare time. After nearly a year, the cording finally settled down, however, I was still having to massage the tissue surrounding the right chest wall.

Before the surgery for the first mastectomy, my surgeon Dr. Kamyab had asked me if she could perform an Axillary clearance. Having never heard or known of this procedure until this time, I agreed. The outcome of that procedure has been, for me, constant worry about Lymphoedema developing in my right arm. Lymphoedema can occur when the lymph nodes are missing or impaired due to surgery and can cause swelling in the affected limb as the lymph fluid builds up in the tissue. I have also read that having Rheumatoid Arthritis can also increase the risk of developing Lymphoedema. I have also been encouraged to use only the left arm for blood tests and also for blood pressure taking. Before every subsequent operation, I had to let the nurses know which arm to use for the cannula and drip and blood pressure cuff.

After the first post-op visit, I was seen by the physiotherapist after every visit to the breast clinic. Shortly after the operation, measurements of my arm were taken, to fit me for a compression sleeve to assist in the prevention of Lymphoedema. These sleeves apply the correct amount of pressure to assist lymph drainage in the right direction and help with circulation. I have seen a case of Lymphoedema and I never want it to happen to me. I wear the sleeve whenever I start to feel tightness or stabbing pain in my arm and also have to massage underneath my arm and around the side of the chest wall quite regularly, otherwise, I can feel the fluid building up under the skin. The physio taught me how to perform a manual lymph drainage massage so I could do it myself at home.

I have also seen a Lymphoedema therapist

since the operations and have purchased a heavy duty compression sleeve and glove, which I wear whenever I travel on an aircraft. As there are long periods of inactivity and reduced cabin pressure when you fly, this can put increased pressure on the lymphatic system. It is really uncomfortable to wear both of these garments. When we flew to Greece and had an eleven-hour flight to Abu Dhabi, I was so ready to get both garments off after we landed. I also wear compression stockings when we fly, to lessen my risk of developing a DVT (Deep vein thrombosis). I also find it very difficult to sleep on flights, as I don't want to sit for very long without moving, again due to the increased risk of both Lymphoedema and DVT. I get up and go for a walk and do some stretching exercises at least every two hours on a long flight, so it's another aspect of my life that has been affected, but one that I will do religiously. Albeit, not always with a big smile on my face, sometimes more like a grimace.

Now that I had had seventeen lymph nodes removed from the right armpit, I had to make sure I didn't do anything that would compromise the lymphatic system. As it is the lymphatic system that helps rid infection from your body, if

I received an injury to the right arm, this could increase my chances of Lymphoedema happening. To take extra care of my arm it was now suggested that I wear gloves when gardening, use rubber gloves when doing the dishes and make sure the water was not too hot, spas were probably not a good idea, as the body can get overheated, not wear clothing which was too tight and cover my skin when in the sun, so I didn't get sunburned. Now I should really only have blood tests taken from my left arm and blood pressure taken there as well. This again lessens the chances of the immune system thinking it is under attack by infection. I wasn't aware of any of these things before the surgery. I may have read about them but I certainly couldn't remember any of them. As my immune system was already compromised due to having Rheumatoid Arthritis, I would have to be extra vigilant. My life hasn't been affected to any great degree, but it's still foremost in my mind when I'm wanting to do any of the things listed.

The three rounds of chemotherapy treatment that I had after the first mastectomy, affected my period cycle. I had read before the chemo started that if a person is near the age of menopause or perimenopause that sometimes the symptoms of menopause can start. I had had a menstrual period in July 2013 and I started my chemo treatment in August 2013. I then didn't have another period until I visited my regular doctor for my annual health checks in June 2014. I think with the internal examination for the Pap smear, it somehow triggered something, and within a week or so it started and was the heaviest I had had for many years.

After June 2014, my period never returned and shortly afterward I was bombarded with the symptoms of menopause! Hot flushes beyond belief, that were so frequent and hot, at times I would cry with frustration. I would have a lovely shower and the minute I got out, my body would just heat up and I would have to find something to fan myself with.

Even now, if I am in a room without some form of air movement, I will have a flush. Needless to say, my handbag has a hand fan in it and I try to remember to take it with me wherever I go. If I don't have one, I will look around for the nearest piece of paper to fan myself with.

My sleep patterns are also affected in a big way. Having hot flushes and night sweats during the night can often wake me up; kicking away the covers and laying like a starfish while pulling the pillow out from under my head. Luckily I wear my birthday suit to bed, otherwise, I'd be ripping clothes off as well. It's one less thing to think of.

The menopausal symptoms sometimes affect the physical closeness between Martin and myself. We try and have a cuddle once we're in bed, but it usually doesn't last long. That's in summer or winter. Martin's a hotty anyway, so put his hot body next to mine and you've got a furnace! We now have a quick cuddle then its "Ok, on your side," and kick the covers off. No spooning for us.

Another very personal issue that arose from the onset of menopause was vaginal dryness. I had never suffered from any problems in that way at any other stage of my life. It's not an issue you expect to have when you're only forty-five years old. Yet we found ourselves in this position and I took it rather personally! It didn't matter how much foreplay we indulged in, I was still left with a hooha as dry as the Simpson Desert. I used to get very upset when I started to feel uncomfortable before and during sex and Martin would tell me that I was dry and I would cry and get angry and say "It's not my fault." We started off using some moisturiser to help things along, but we knew that wasn't really the best thing to be using. My husband was so understanding during this time. I'm sure he was feeling the stress also on an intimate level, but he never made me feel as if it was my fault.

After probably six to eight months and with a lot of support from my gorgeous hubby, I was finally able to get over myself and ask for help. I just decided that if this was how it was going to be, then like the flushes, I would have to adapt my way of living. When I saw my regular doctor after this decision, I discussed the problems I was having and she recommended a lubricant which she said other menopausal women had had good results with. Later at the chemist, we looked at all the different lubricants and bought a couple of different ones to try. I found that some stung my bits, while others were sticky, which was just as bad. We finally hit on a product which was recommended through a party plan business for adult romance and related products. This product is called Pure Pleasure Signature and it is a silicone based lubricant. It is available to order from the Pure Romance website or one of their party plan consultants. And it is amazing!!! All I can say folks, is try and get help for these symptoms sooner rather than later. You will save yourselves and your relationship a lot of grief. Using this product is now our 'normal', so if Martin happens to say "Hun, you need something," I just head to the bedside drawer and get my wonderful helper out and let the fun begin!

To help with the onset of menopause, I visited the Menopause clinic at King Edward Memorial Hospital (who knew there was one there!!) and had two visits with the doctors there in 2013 and 2014. Unfortunately, the first drug I was advised to take Gabapentin, did not agree with me and I developed light headedness and dizziness. After a quick phone call, the nurse recommended stopping the medication. We tried another medication Endep, but after three months I decided I would just try to cope as best I could, without the extra stress of another medication in my body. I didn't really feel that the medication was helping. Since then, I have learned, as every other menopausal woman does, to live with my hot body!! I no longer get upset, I just grab my fan or the nearest item I can find and fan away until the flush subsides.

I recently visited the menopause clinic again in late 2018, after a referral from Dr. Ponniah, to see if there were any new treatment options that I could look into. I am currently taking a medication called Catapres which I am hoping will reduce the symptoms, but only time will tell.

The doctor at the menopause clinic also asked me if I had heard of CBT (Cognitive behaviour therapy). I said that I had and we discussed some studies that are now being done into how CBT can help menopausal women. I was also given some reading material on the subject and have found it very interesting. I found that I have been using many of the strategies included in the material throughout the years since the chemotherapy.

When I started with the hot flushes I would get upset and angry which may have increased the intensity of the flush. Over the years I have taught myself to just go with it, fan myself and breathe deeply and wait until it passes. Even when I'm in a plane or restaurant, which are places with little or no air circulation and I start to have a flush I just stay calm and go through it. The strange looks I get sometimes I find quite funny. Often I will have a staff member approach and ask me if I'm feeling okay and I just reply "Yes, just having a flush, it'll be over in a minute." It has now become a part of my life and so I learn to deal with it, in the best way I can. Again, I will say that seeking help earlier rather than later may assist with the symptoms and spare you a lot of grief. What works for some, will not for others and vice-versa. So give it a go.

Along with the onset of menopause, the chemotherapy also made my body hair fall out, although I did choose to shave my hair off before it fell out. This decision was easy, however, when my hair started to grow back, it came through silver and black.

I had been dyeing my hair for many years, and I had mentioned to Martin many times of the hassle I felt it was, let alone the cost. I used to say to him "If I could just see what colour it would be if I cut it all short and then just let it grow and see." You really do have to watch what you wish for. Anyway, my funky hair started to grow and by December 2013 I had a little short crop that I would put a little bit of mousse in. I had this hairstyle for about six months. I used to get all positive compliments. One of my customers at the foreign exchange used to say "You're rocking that hairstyle, Caroline." This lady had also had breast cancer and told me that before her cancer she had had dead straight hair. After her treatment was completed and her hair grew back, it came through afro curly. That got me wondering then, what I would end up with. After six months of being grey, I finally tired of it. When I sat at work and looked out the front doors, the only people I saw who had my hair colour were elderly. I had had enough.

Luckily for me, my daughter Jade was completing a Certificate two in hairdressing. So, I indulged in all of the discounted hair treatments that I could. I started feeling much better about myself when I finally saw myself in the mirror and I didn't look old anymore. I didn't have a haircut for four years, besides a tiny trim. I knew what I had lost and I didn't want to lose it again. My hair grew rather long over this time (see below) and did become a little bit hard to handle.

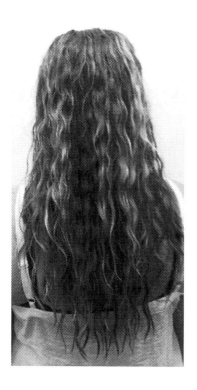

The first time I went to a salon for my first haircut, the young lady kept asking me if I was sure that I wanted to cut it. By this stage, I had come to the conclusion that it was only hair, after all, and I knew it would grow back. Again, I don't think I was ready until this time to do it.

As well as losing the hair on my head, I also lost most of my eyelashes, which I only realised when I put mascara on to attend Jade's year twelve graduation and saw I had about five lashes on each side! My eyebrows were still not bad, however, every now and again I would touch them up with some eyeliner. My arm and leg hair seemed less affected and stayed pretty much normal throughout the treatment. My pubic region though became as bald as a badger.

I said to Martin "You better enjoy this, as this is the only time it's going to look like this!"

He thought that was hilarious. You've got to see the positives in every situation, no bikini line shaving for some time. I can't actually remember the hair falling out in that area, but I think I had other things on my mind. It took a good while for all the hair to grow back. And I'm happy to say, I was lucky enough to have it all grow back, just as it was before the treatment.

After the second mastectomy, I had the expanders put in straight away. So after the operation, I came home minus a large breast, no nipples at all, but I had two small lumps on my chest as the expanders had each had one hundred mills put in them. As I mentioned in the last chapter, these expanders were not the most attractive objects. My chest looked square and again I felt most unattractive. It was good to finally be even in my clothing, but everything I wore looked horrible. As I ended up having them in for just under two years, I hadn't bought any new clothes as everything I tried on looked awful. I didn't wear any nice tops in summer as I felt my chest looked unattractive. I mostly wore t-shirts or long flowing shirts that would cover me well.

I became even more self-conscious around Martin after this operation. We had at least had the left breast for a few more months after the first mastectomy, but now we were left with nothing. It was so weird to hug Martin and feel parts of our bodies' touch that hadn't touched before, due to my big boobs being in the way. I tried not to look in the mirror after showering as at first, it was quite shocking. I definitely didn't feel like a woman. I knew I was comfortable with the decision I had made to remove the remaining breast. Until it happens though, you don't know how it will affect you. As always my wonderful hubby tried his best to allay my fears and told me often how beautiful I was. Easy to hear, but hard to believe. Please be gentle with yourself or your loved one, it's a hard time and we all react differently to gestures made and words spoken.

During the time we had to wait for the implant exchange operation, I guess I just got used to having my body in the state it was in. Martin's encouragement would have also been a catalyst for my acceptance of my body at that time. So it gradually became a bit easier to look at my reflection in the mirror without judgement and to not feel as self-conscious, when we were having some fun in the bedroom.

I did look after my scars every day, which is quite important, by applying Bio Oil. I would have my shower and then gently massage a small amount of this oil onto the scars on both sides of my body. I also regularly massaged the sides of my chest as the scarring while not seen, was definitely there under the skin. The scars on my chest became quite faded by the time I had the exchange surgery. I must admit, I haven't been as good with this since the last operation and I can see the difference in the colour of the scars.

Earlier in this chapter, I mentioned the ongoing dread of cancer coming back somewhere in my body. As I had started menopause brought on by the surgery and/or chemotherapy, I discussed with Martin my desire to have my ovaries taken out. If there was something I could do to decrease my risk of having ovarian cancer, then I wanted in. I saw my regular doctor and discussed my thoughts with her and after the consultation, she gave me a referral to a gynaecologist. I received an appointment in April 2015.

I went along to the appointment and talked with the doctor about my reasons for wanting the operation. She let me know about the procedure and possible side effects from having it done. I told her I had researched the outcomes and I didn't feel they were any worse than what I was currently experiencing. I told her I would do everything I could to look after my body following the operation. I had to undergo an ultrasound before the operation, to make sure everything was where it should be. The gynaecologist told me that if the fallopian tubes were all in good condition that she would take them as well as the ovaries, and I told her I thought that would be a good idea. I also told her that Martin and I were going on holidays to Melbourne, Uluru (Ayers Rock) and Sydney in July, so the operation would not be scheduled for those dates. When I received the letter from the hospital with the date of the operation, I quickly called and spoke to someone regarding the proximity of the operation to the start of our holidays. I received a call from one of the nurses later that day, who let me know that I would probably be fine to fly out the week after the operation.

I had a Laparoscopic Bilateral Salpingo-Oophorectomy or Laparoscopic BSO on the 2nd July 2015. The operation went smoothly and I stayed overnight as I had a catheter in, and went home the next day, happy as Larry. I could at least cross one cancer of my list, which for my peace of mind was very important. I haven't noticed any subsequent issues arising from the BSO. I make sure I take a Vitamin D and Calcium tablet every day and try to look after my physical health as well as I can.

During the week following the operation, I had only mild stiffness in my shoulder blades. This was a result of the gas that was pumped into my body. I took it easy during this week and on the 10th July, Martin and I flew out for our whirlwind holiday. We went camel riding while in Uluru, but as it was not a jolting ride, my body handled it beautifully. I enjoyed my holiday immensely. This operation was a great decision for me.

Having the second mastectomy was not really

a big decision for me. My desire to continue living far outweighed the loss of my breasts. Now, more than five years later, my thoughts remain the same, as to the reason for doing it. But… I miss the feel of my natural breasts every day. When I take my clothes off at night there is no fall to my breasts, no slight movement. Martin will look at me out of the corner of his eyes with a grin on his face, and I know he's watching me, but I also know what he's seeing. I don't see them as breasts anymore. They don't look like real breasts and from inside my body, they don't feel like real breasts. Don't get me wrong. My surgeon did the most amazing work with them.

But this is where it gets quite tough. Parts of my body, my breasts that I fed my children with, (unsuccessfully though it may have been) that I identified with as a woman, no longer look or feel how they have for the past thirty-five years. I miss them. The softness and shape of them. How the nipple would react to the cold or stimulation. Now, there is firmness. No reaction of my newly formed nipples to the cold or stimulation. No feeling in them at all in fact, or to most of the skin on my chest. I know when Martin is touching them, by the feeling of pressure on the chest. The shape of one of my new little nipples didn't last and now looks like a melted puddle of nipple. It's the age old saying "You don't know what you have, till it's gone." I used to complain about how saggy my breasts were, how being pregnant and gaining then losing weight had affected them. They were really heading 'down south'. I know it's not the actual breasts I miss, it's the feeling that the breasts gave me. The sensuality and excitement associated with touching and stimulating them. The objects on my chest now, don't allow me to feel stimulation and they certainly don't make me feel sensual. I have yet to have the areola tattooed on them to complete the look, but even then I'm sure, it will be purely cosmetic. They might look more like natural breasts, but they will still feel firm and unmoving. I don't have much fatty tissue left in either breast and as the implants are under the pectoral muscle, the feeling of the breast is possibly firmer than someone else who may have had breast enhancement, within the existing fatty tissue of their breast.

I could have explored the possibility of having a reconstruction using my own fat and tissue, using a flap technique. Either a TRAM flap which utilises abdominal muscles and fatty tissue, or a DIEP flap which uses fatty stomach tissue and skin. Or even a Latissmus Dorsi flap (using the Latissmus Dorsi muscle, located on the back under the armpit and beneath the shoulder blade); some fat, muscle and blood vessels are used to help create the new breast. I chose not to use these options, as I had read that as with any tissue transplant, sometimes the tissue can become necrotic. I didn't want something else to happen which would set back my recovery. Little did any of us know at the time, that I would have to endure another operation when capsular contracture developed with the first set of implants. I feel though, that my recovery time with the implant operation would have been a lot quicker, than if I had needed an operation to remove necrotic skin and tissue.

The veins in my left hand after the chemo treatments have never been the same. I used to be a blood donor and donating was always an easy process. I would make sure I drank at least a litre of water before each donation. My veins would be fat and plumped and just waiting to be drained. I generally always used my left arm for donations as I found it more comfortable than my right. After the chemo treatments, the veins in my left hand seemed to become constricted and hard. With all of the surgeries following the initial surgery, the phlebotomists and nurses often had trouble finding veins that were useful.

With one operation, I asked the anaesthetist to put the cannula in my foot, as it was less hassle and less painful for me to have it there, rather than my hand or forearm. In summer, my veins on both hands used to swell and look quite unsightly. Now the veins in my left hand are barely visible even when I am hot. With my R.A. I have to have a blood test every three months and I stress every time, in case the girls have difficulty finding a vein. As I mentioned earlier, the right arm was pretty much now out of bounds for any procedure due to the Lymphoedema risk.

I mentioned briefly in chapter two that when having chemotherapy some people lose weight, while others can gain weight. Well lucky me, I gained weight. Bugger. During the four rounds of chemo spread out over three months, I gained about three kilos. My face became really bloated and I felt a bit like a water balloon. All squishy and soft. It's funny that I put on weight as I hardly ate for every one out of three weeks. But I think it was the drugs and that it was just a side effect of having them in my system. It was sometimes hard to deal with, as my body was going through changes anyway with the mastectomies. To then start putting on weight without the joy of eating lots of yummy things, did make me feel a bit sad every now and again.

Speaking of weight gain, I also put some weight on before the surgeries even started. If I'm honest, and okay folks I will be, I believe I put on maybe five to six kilos during the time from diagnosis to when the chemo started. So from May to August. I just threw caution to the wind. I told Martin that as I didn't know whether I was going to live or die if I wanted a triple choc muffin and a large hot chocolate, then I was going to have it. And enjoy it! And I did!

Just after the chemo finished I started taking Tamoxifen. Weight gain is not usually listed as a side effect of Tamoxifen, although I have seen a lot of posts on breast cancer websites from women saying they believe that Tamoxifen has caused their weight gain. I believe for me, it was a combination of many things that have caused me to gain weight throughout the years since diagnosis.

My pre-treatment weight gain was due to

eating whatever I wanted. This was then added to, during the chemo cycle. Martin and I used to walk quite regularly around our suburb, however, as I had each operation, whereby I needed time to heal and convalesce, these walks became less and less. This fact would have contributed to my weight gain also.

Now that I'm smack bang in the menopause phase, I suppose I could try and blame that for being the cause behind my stagnant weight loss and 'mummy tummy'. I will admit though, that up till now, I haven't tried very hard to lose the weight. But, as I said to Martin recently, if I'm not doing anything to help myself, then the weight will not fall off on its own.

I am probably ten plus, kilos heavier than before my diagnosis. So, this year for my birthday I asked Martin to get me a gym membership for twelve months. It's been a bit stop-start, but I'm not too hard on myself if I don't go, particularly on work days. I know that all the research says that I should maintain a healthy weight to decrease my risk of a large number of medical conditions. I will do my best. If you understand the 'traffic light food system', then I am trying to cut out the 'red foods', eat sparingly of the 'orange foods' and enjoy a lot of the 'green foods'. So hang in there, if the kilos have gone on. Concentrate on one thing at a time. And be gentle on yourself.

On thinking about the cancer diagnosis, I couldn't remember anyone on my mum's side of the family ever having had breast cancer and neither could mum. On dad's side, however, there were a couple of cases. I learned from my aunt Marion that two of my great, great aunts had breast cancer and sadly both had passed from this disease. My aunty Valma also had an encapsulated tumour removed, and had one round of chemotherapy treatment. Aunt Marion herself also had a breast cancer diagnosis in 2014, which resulted in a mastectomy on the right side. As I had to share some history with my surgeons before and during my treatment regime, this information obviously got one of them thinking about things.

So it happened that during my initial treatment, one of my surgeons made a referral to a company called Genetic Services of W.A. This company accepts referrals for patients who are at increased risk of cancer. They have a program called the Familial Cancer Program, which can provide testing for inherited cancer predisposition conditions, such as breast and ovarian (BRCA1 and 2). I was contacted by the company and provided my health record and also a family tree, on which I had to state if the relative had suffered from any form of cancer and if they were alive or deceased. From this information, a determination would be made as to my suitability for free genetic testing (covered by Medicare). From the information I supplied, it was concluded that I was not in a high-risk category. The risk factor is calculated as a percentage and as I was under the required percentage, genetic testing would not be offered. I was told, however, to be mindful of the family and my own history and to remind family members to have regular check-ups.

I updated the information in subsequent years after losing some family members to cancer. This updated information raised the risk percentage for me and I was contacted by a geneticist from the company in 2018. I had a consultation with the geneticist, and at the end of the discussion, she offered me the testing and told me the cost would be covered by Medicare. The testing was as simple as a blood test, which I had performed later that day and the samples were sent off for testing. There were five particular genetic mutations which my samples were tested for. These included BRCA 1 and BRCA 2. I was told that if the results did not show as positive, the outcome may be termed as inconclusive.

My results, which I received in a letter about six weeks later, were in that category. This result meant that I did not have the BRCA 1 or 2 mutation, or the other three that I had been tested for. The inconclusive result meant that I may/may not have a mutation in one of the other many hundreds of mutations that can occur, which is why the result is not termed negative. I was really happy to have received this result. I felt better knowing I did not have this gene mutation, and it was great to share this information with my family. I try to encourage my family to be very vigilant about their health, as I know first-hand that early detection can give a much better outcome.

On nearing completion of this memoir, I made a decision. I had not asked my family for any actual input, in other words, I just included them. However, I realised that their words may offer some insight for others going through the same experience. So I asked Jade and my mum to give me something I could include. I told them I knew it might be hard and possibly confrontational for them. We have never discussed what we all went through. It's like it happened, and that was that. So, the following paragraphs are the words of some of my beautiful family;

My mum's words;

"Words a mother never wants to hear, is their child has a life-threatening illness. It's hard to put into words all the emotions that hit you - it's not real - it's not happening. Your stomach turns, your vision blurs. But you say to yourself it's going to be alright. That your child's a fighter and they have come a long way in the treatment of breast cancer. There, I've said the words that make me cry. That is what my daughter had to endure to come out safe at the other end. Also, not forgetting the prayers that were said daily and often. Thank God for my daughter."

Jade's words;

"I'd just come home from celebrating finishing my year 12 exams with some friends when mum messaged me asking me to come home. On arriving, everyone was seated in the lounge (mum, Martin, Tyson, and Nan) I knew that whatever was going to be said- it wasn't going to be good. That's when mum told Tyson and I that she had breast cancer. Instantly I thought about the worst case scenario - becoming an adult without my mum to guide me.

To be honest, the way I dealt with what my mum went through was to stick my head in the sand and ignore what was happening. For me, it was easier than dealing with it - seeing her look so sick in bed and watching her whole body change. The only thing I didn't ignore was the day that Martin and I sat out the back of the house with mum while Martin shaved all her hair off. That was something I knew I wouldn't be able to cope with if I just saw the before and after - I had to see the progression.

When asked to write how mums cancer affected me, I kept drawing blanks. What should I say? What did I do to help her through it? I wasn't like Martin who held mums hand through every appointment, every surgery, and every breakdown because of how hard it all was. I wasn't like Nanna who helped anywhere she could, as support, or to take care of me and my brother. What did I do?

I didn't do enough. When a family member goes through cancer, everyone reacts differently. If I were to go back, I definitely would've wanted to be there as more support - helped more around the house, to take the weight off Martin. Listened more to what mum was going through, instead of blocking out whatever she said. I just wish I was there for my mum who has always been there for me."

After Jade sent me the words that she wanted to be included in the book, I sent her back a message. I told her that both she and Tyson had helped us, by sticking together, loving each other and not giving us an ounce of trouble during the experience. I also told her that on reflecting on her words, maybe Martin and I should have asked them to help around the house. It may have helped them to feel like they were a part of what was happening and not separate to it. I don't remember if I asked the children how they were feeling throughout the five years. I think I just accepted that they were okay, as there were no outward signs that they were feeling anything other than fine. It was enough for me during that time to see them doing their best at school, supporting each other and being able to smile. As I said to Jade, it's not always about doing something physical, like the dishes. What I saw, was worth a years worth of dishes.

If I have any last words to offer that we found

helpful, they would be to try and keep loving and laughing during the experience. I've often told people when sharing our experience, that it was easy for me to be happy and smiling most of the time, as we had received a good diagnosis and my outcome looked good. For those facing a different battle, humour may be the last thing on their mind, so please be mindful of saying things that are not helpful. It's always wise to remember the saying "Walk a mile in my shoes", before offering your well-meaning advice. Be gentle with yourself or your loved one in body, mind, and spirit. Be honest with the communication about how YOU feel and what YOU need and want. Research your options, either by talking to your doctor or a reputable organisation such as, in W.A, Cancer Council of W.A. or Breast Cancer Care W.A. Reach out if you need support on any level. There are many people out there with the skills and knowledge to help you. Just allow them the opportunity to enter your life.

Martin's perspective on Re-building

Having read through everything that Caroline has written a few things really stand out. The first is how incredible it is that we (I will talk more about this later) have gone through this whole journey with all of its ups and downs and, I believe, have an even stronger relationship now than when all of this started. Caroline mentioned quite a few times that she had been worried about how I would see her with all of the changes that she has gone through. I have thought about this a lot and can't remember ever thinking that I wanted her less because of anything she had been through, or anything that had been removed, or anything that had been replaced. She is still my beautiful wife no matter what.

The second thing is the word we. One thing I want anyone reading this to realise is that we both went through this. I know I didn't suffer through any of the physical stuff but I do know that is has taken a toll on me mentally. I don't care how tough anyone thinks they are, seeing someone you love go through this is hard and it does have an effect on you. As I mentioned in the first chapter I was offered the chance to talk to someone but didn't take it up. Do I regret that I don't know? Will I take up the opportunity if offered to me again, I don't know but probably would. Please don't let yourself get in the way. What can you lose? Maybe, just maybe you might find it beneficial.

Another thing to consider is the effect it has on those around you. Family, friends and even workmates. This disease is very confrontational and a lot of people don't know how to react or what to say when you tell them. Understand this, when people react in different ways. I am sure it is just their coping mechanism kicking into high gear.

The third thing that stands out to me, is how incredible it is that Caroline kept such comprehensive records about appointments, operations and who she had spoken too and when. I can tell you I would not have kept any records and would never have even considered writing this. Just another example of what an amazing woman she is.

One more thing. Little reminders can be upsetting. I have obviously read what Caroline has written. This has resulted in tears and laughter.

The thing that upsets me the most, is any photo of Caroline with no hair. Her scars don't affect me the way seeing her with no hair does. I don't know why this upsets me to the extent it does, but it does. Even writing this is hard and bringing a tear to my eye. There is a photo in this book and I know I will struggle every time I look at it.

Time to get a bit personal. I am sure our children (we both have two from previous relationships) if they read some parts of this book, may have cause for some sleepless nights but welcome to our nightmare. The whole 'dryness thing' was a real issue for me. Not the physical aspect but what it did to me mentally. I started thinking that maybe Caroline did not find me attractive anymore and that I did not turn her on. It did start to affect me physically (I am sure you know what I mean) which only made things worse for both of us in the state of mind that we were in. Luckily it was something we worked through and have come out of the other end with no further problems in this area. Just a bit of understanding, communication, and patience have returned the ledger to credit if you know what I mean.

Caroline's fake boobies are something we are both coming to terms with. I know she has no sensation in them so it does stop me from touching them during special cuddle time. Why? It is sort of like having a shower with a raincoat on. Yes, you are in the shower but is it really going to have the desired effect? This might be hard for most to understand. It is hard for me to understand. As mentioned I do catch a sneaky look at them whenever the opportunity presents itself. Why? Well, they are my wife's boobs. I am sure any husband would do the same thing. And they're pretty good looking to boot.

So what I have I gained from all of this? Many things come to mind but a few really stand out. In our case, how strong it has made our relationship. We are lucky there. This sort of thing has ended a lot of relationships. It is too much for some people to cope with. Also, how strong it has made me. I look at life differently now. I have never been a negative person but I believe now I have an even more positive outlook on life.

Going forward from this we have decided to live life the best that we can. What do I mean by this? We are living in the moment and planning on being here for a long time. We have dreams and ambitions for the future but we know that it can be taken away, so we don't waste a second. I suggested some years ago that we take a certain trip for our 50th birthdays. I was told that we were not going to wait and went on that holiday the next year. We are lucky to be in the position we are and will not let the grass grow under our feet, until we have too.

Printed in the United States
By Bookmasters